NEW PARADIGMS FOR
SHANG HAN LUN

Integrating Korean Sasang Constitutional
Medicine and Japanese Kampo Medicine

ANGIE KIM, PH.D., L.AC.

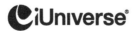

NEW PARADIGMS FOR SHANG HAN LUN
INTEGRATING KOREAN SASANG CONSTITUTIONAL MEDICINE AND JAPANESE KAMPO MEDICINE

iUniverse books may be ordered through booksellers or by contacting:

iUniverse
1663 Liberty Drive
Bloomington, IN 47403
www.iuniverse.com
1-800-Authors (1-800-288-4677)

Because of the dynamic nature of the Internet, any web addresses or links contained in this book may have changed since publication and may no longer be valid. The views expressed in this work are solely those of the author and do not necessarily reflect the views of the publisher, and the publisher hereby disclaims any responsibility for them.

Any people depicted in stock imagery provided by Thinkstock are models, and such images are being used for illustrative purposes only. Certain stock imagery © Thinkstock.

ISBN: 978-1-5320-1813-8 (sc)
ISBN: 978-1-5320-1814-5 (e)

Print information available on the last page.

iUniverse rev. date: 03/30/2017

Table of Contents

Foreword

Studying Traditional Asian Medicine is like the blind men touching a giant elephant to learn what it is like. With thousands years of history, there is a myriad of literature and theories, and not only is it hard to perceive the big picture, it takes effort to distinguish between the gems and pebbles.

As a practitioner, it is also very easy to be stuck in one outstanding theory and delude oneself that he or she has mastered the whole Traditional Asian Medicine. However, Traditional Asian Medicine itself is a masterpiece that has not been completed.

Here are two pieces of a picture of the giant elephant of Traditional Asian Medicine that have been practiced in China, Korea, and Japan but not fully adopted in traditional Asian medical education in the US.

These two can be indicators in prescribing formulas based on *Shang Han Lun*, one from the individual constitutional perspective of Dr. Lee Jema and the other from the single herbal functional perspective of Dr. Todo Yoshimas. I believe these are crucial clues to putting all the pieces together in Asian herbal formula practice, yet need to be further studied and proved in clinical settings.

My clinical case studies are also added after the introduction of Dr. Lee and Dr. Todo's studies. These clinical cases are the little fruits of my ten years of practice after struggling to find better way to approach to Asian Medicine. I hope this book can provide herbal practitioners with stepping stones on the journey to mastering Asian Medicine.

Angie Kim,Ph.D., L.Ac.

About the Author

Angie Kim

Angie Kim has practiced acupuncture and traditional Asian herbal medicine in California since 2005. Her vision is to contribute herself to the development of traditional Asian Medicine by healing people in the most natural way and sharing her knowledge and experience with others.

Angie holds a doctorate in Traditional Asian Medicine. On graduating Summa Cum Laude from Emperor's College of Traditional Oriental Medicine, she has taken her continuing trainings including Korean Medicine Program at Kyung Hee University of South Korea, Korean Sasang Constitutional Medicine Program with Dr. Man Hur who is the third generation Sasang Medicine practitioner, and studies of Shang Han Lun and Jin Gui Yao Lue with great Korean Medicine scholars.

She also lectured at Dongguk University in Los Angeles and School of Alternative Medicine, Life University in Gardena, California. Now her passion is to share her clinical experience of Sasang Constitutional Medicine and Shang Han Lun with peer acupuncturists and herbalists all over the world.

Chapter 1

Korean Constitutional Medicine

An American author, Lierre Keith, published a book titled "The Vegetarian Myth" in 2009 revealing the risk of a vegan diet after she suffered from numerous chronic health problems and decided that the vegan diet she had followed for twenty years was to blame. People on nutritional diet websites or blogs have been debating this book, arguing which diet is better, vegetarian or non- vegetarian.

When we get to know about body constitution, we don't have to struggle to pick one diet or another as an answer for everyone. When we fully understand that there are different body types and corresponding diets for each, it is a lot easier to understand how our bodies work.

While some people become healthier and lose weight with a vegetarian diet, some don't. Others state that they have had great results from the Atkins diet, a low carbohydrate diet focusing on the consumption of meat for weight loss, originally promoted by Dr. Robert C. Atkins, who wrote a best- selling book about the diet in 1972.

Most people seem to vaguely understand that there is no one diet that works for everyone and no one herbal formula or medicine that works for everyone, even people with the same issues, but not a lot of people seem to fully understand body constitution, which is the key factor in deciding each person's diet and supplement intake.

In the history of Western Medicine, the Greek physician Hippocrates(460-370 BC) introduced the Four Temperament theory and Galen(AD129-200) developed it further, searching for physiological reasons for different behaviors in humans.

However, modern medical science has rejected the theory, and it is only used as a metaphor within certain psychological fields.

In Eastern Medical history, Ayurvedic medicine in India and Sasang Constitutional Medicine(SCM) in Korea were developed and are still being practiced actively today. Especially, SCM fleshed out the ideas of different body types in Nei Jing[1] (475BC-260AD) although it expanded and differed on the grouping of each body type, giving more detailed information.

In Chapter 72 of *LingShu* of Nei Jing, the concept of constitution was first mentioned as five different body types. Based on an analysis of old medical literature, Dr. Lee Je-ma(1836-1900), a Korean Traditional Eastern Medicine practitioner, postulated the theory of SCM. He indicated that, among the five body types described in the Nei Jing (Greater Yang type, Lesser Yang type, Greater Yin type, Lesser Yin type and Yin-Yang balanced type), the Yin–Yang balanced type, which was described as a perfect human type, did not exist. Moreover, this classification was not practical for treatment.[2]

The philosophy of SCM was developed by Dr. Lee, in his book 'Dongui Suse Bowon(東醫「世保元)' in 1894. Sasang(四象) means 'Four shapes' or 'Four Images', which shows that one of the basic ideas of Dr. Lee is 'internal energy, external shape (氣裏形表)[3]', meaning internal energy is manifested externally. Based on this concept, four different body types were identified. Those are Tai Yang(Greater Yang), Shao Yang(Lesser Yang), Tai Yin(Greater Yin), and Shao Yin(Lesser Yin), which will be explained later in detail.

---

[1] Huang Di Nei Jing (皇帝內經): The Emperor's Inner Canon. It is an ancient Chinese Medical text that has been treated as the fundamental doctrinal source for Chinese medicine for more than two millennia.

[2] Dr. Song Il-Byung, <An introduction to Sasang Constitutional Medicine> Seoul: Jipmoondang International, 2005

[3] The theory of 'internal energy, external shape (氣裏形表)' is from Dr. Heo Jun's 'Dongui Bogam (東醫寶鑑)'.
Dongui Bogam is traditional Korean Medicine book compiled by Dr. Heo and is on UNESCO's Memory of the World Programme as of July 2009.

Dr. Song Il-Byung, a Traditional Eastern Medicine doctor and professor in Kyung Hee university in Korea reinterpreted the Sasang philosophy in comparison with the one in Nei Jing, stating;

"The philosophy of the Nei Jing is based on the belief that everything is classified into Five primary substances (wood, fire, earth, metal, water). Compared with the Nei Jing, the philosophy of Sasang medicine believes that 'Things exist, Principles exist' and 'Human mind, Human body' on top of a system that groups things into four images. Through this introduction of a new philosophy, Sasang medicine could set up four constitutions, each with its own body-shape and physiology and pathology of the internal organs."[4]

As Dr. Lee wrote in his book, the division of these 4 constitutions originated from the Nei Jing. However, it has to be pointed out that his creative thinking about the division into four constitutions is due to the relative functional size of the organs, which is a remarkable idea in the history of Eastern Medicine.[5] This is also the first approach based on the Yin and Yang theory[6] that focused on individual difference rather than the difference of the pathological symptoms.

Although these 4 terms of Tai Yang, Tai Yin, Shao Yang, and Shao Yin may sound familiar, since they are also used in the 6 channel theory of Shang Han Lun[7], the actual concepts are completely different in that Shang Han Lun described them as the stages of disease progression not as body types. These 4 constitutional terminologies are also different from the ones in I Ching[8] since these 4 images are described as basic units of all things and cannot be divided further whereas in I Ching they are produced from yin and yang and can be further divided into the Eight Trigrams (Ba Gua 八卦).

---

[4] Dr. Song Il-Byung, <Basic Principles of SaSang Medicine>

[5] Dr. Kang Joobong, <The dynamics of Shang Han Lun>, published by IOMRI

[6] This is one of the basic theories in Traditional Eastern Medicine, which represent opposite but complementary qualities. It is also a basic concept of classical Chinese science and philosophy and a central principle of different forms of martial arts.

[7] Known in English as 'The treatise on Cold injury'. Is a Chinese medical treatise that was compiled by Dr. Zhang ZhongJing sometime before the year 220. Is amongst the oldest complete clinical textbooks in the world.

[8] The Classic of Changes(易經). Ancient divination text and the oldest chinese classics. Part of the Five Classics

In the article *Sasang Constitutional Medicine as a Holistic Tailored Medicine*, Dr. Lee's unique idea of the 4 constitutional organ system is well described.

"An explanation of internal visceral systems, SCM uses the same terminology found in TCM (Traditional Chinese Medicine), but each creates a different system of classification. SCM regards the heart as the king among the five viscera, which is equivalent to the mind. Departing from the visceral theory in TCM, where viscera are assigned in pairs, zang and fu, SCM assumes a theory of visceral groups: the lung, kidney, liver and spleen groups. The lung group includes the lungs, tongue, esophagus region, ears, brain and skin. The spleen group consists of the spleen, stomach, breasts, eyes and tendons. The constituents of the liver group are the liver, small intestine, nose, lumbar region and muscles. The kidney group has the kidney, large intestine, urethra, bladder, mouth and bones. Among these groups, it is believed that specific inter-regulatory relations are present between specific pairs of visceral group. As such, visceral groups are classified into two pairs: one consists of the spleen and the kidney group and the other is composed of the lung and the liver group. The relation in each pair of visceral groups is akin to the balancing state of a seesaw. In this respect, a hyperactive state in one group leads to a relatively deficient state in its counterpart. The state of hyperactivity in the lung group leads to a hypoactive state of the liver in Tai Yang types, but vice versa in Tai Yin types. Finally, the state of hyperactivity in the spleen group leads to a hypoactive state of the kidney group in Shao Yang types, but vice versa in Shao Yin types."[9]

Based on the imbalances defined by these inter-regulatory relations, each body type manifests uniquely in terms of appearance, physical traits, mental and emotional characteristics, physiological and pathological signs and symptoms, etc.

Dr. Song, in his book *Sasang Medicine Made Easy*, suggested that constitutional diagnosis should be made comprehensively based on all three of the appearances, the nature of the disposition, and the pathological symptoms. Especially, in the earlier practice of Sasang constitutional medicine, hasty conclusions considering only one or two of these aspects can lead to a wrong diagnosis.

---

[9] Kim Jongyeol and Duong Duc Pham, <Sasang Constitutional Medicine as a Holistic Tailored Medicine>

It is well known among Eastern Herbalists that the right formula determined from the right diagnosis can make a great improvement in a patient's condition but the other way around can not only accomplish nothing but may even make the patient worse. Especially, in Sasang constitutional medical practice, the right formula used for the right person is the key to treat any condition. Although Sasang Constitutional Medicine may not be a perfect system for treating people, it can provide us with main indicators that lead us in the right direction. When herbal practitioners can grasp the idea of grouping the 4 constitutions, they will come a step closer to being able to use not only Sasang constitutional formulas but also any other formulas including Shang Han Lun formulas.

With herbal prescription as the main treatment method of Sasang constitutional Medicine, Dr. Lee Je-Ma thought highly of Dr. Zhang Zhongjing, and quoted many symptom presentations and formulas from Dr. Zhang's Shang Han Lun. However, he described them according to his system of Sasang constitutional theory, not following the 6 Channel theory of Shang Han Lun. He also created his own formulas that he deemed beneficial for each constitution.

Dr. Lee stated in his book that Dr. Zhang's formulas for the three yin stages (Tai Yin, Shao Yin, and Jue Yin) belong to Shao Yin Ren,[10] the formulas for the Shao Yang stage belong to Shao Yang Ren[11], and the formulas for Tai Yang and Yang Ming stages belong to Shao Yang Ren, Shao Yin Ren, and Tai Yin Ren[12], but mostly to Shao Yin Ren. So Dr. Lee concluded that Dr. Zhang invented formulas for Shao Yin Ren almost 100 percent, obtained formulas for Shao Yang Ren about 50 percent, barely for Tai Yin Ren, and none for Tai Yang Ren. Dr. Lee also invented new formulas for the Shao Yang, Tai Yin and Tai Yang constitutions under the influence of famous Chinese doctors in the Song, Yuan, and Ming dynasty.[13]

In herbal formula practices in the US, Dr. Lee's innovative diagnostic methods and new formulas are extremely useful since there are higher percentages of Tai Yin Ren and Tai Yang Ren among non-Asian ethnic groups.

---

[10] A person with Shao Yin constitution
[11] A Person with Shao Yang constitution
[12] A Person with Tai Yin constitutio
[13] Sasang Constitutional Medicine, published by Jip Moon Dang (Korean Version)

1. Shao Yin Constitution

Points of differentiation

Shaoyins usually have a well-developed hip area and a less developed chest area. The lower body is more developed than the upper. The skin tends to be soft and relatively moist. Muscle tone cannot be developed easily for this body type thus generally weak muscles or even sagging muscles in seniors can be found. They tend to hunch forward due to their weak chest area. For the face, the lower jaw is relatively bigger and well developed.

It is said that Shaoyins tend to be petite and have a small physique, but in the US with its variety of ethnic group, there are a variety of Shao Yin body types, some tall and slim, and some are even corpulent. The statue of Venus shows the classic female appearance of a Shao Yin body type, with a smooth body line and soft skin. The feet of this type are usually very cold to the touch due to strong Kidney water energy. People with the Shao Yin body type usually complain of low energy due to weaker Spleen energy, and generally experience an aversion to cold and less perspiration.

Shaoyins have a tendency to introversion and a feminine nature, and are docile, self-possessed, and circumspect. They would rather stay at home than go out, and are always nervous that things might be wrong, even with little things. They are usually detailed oriented and very organized, so they can accomplish goals when they are determined and push ahead with a given project. However, due to their passive attitude and low energy, it is easy for them to get complacent and idle, not being able to overcome obstacles.

All the above physical and mental traits are manifestations originating from organ imbalances of the large kidneys and the small Spleen in Shao Yin body types. The size of organs referred to in SCM original texts means the energetic and functional dimension of the organs, not the actual size of the organs.

People with Shao Yin body types, due to Spleen weakness, tend to have digestive problems when they are not in good condition, so it is said that Shaoyins are healthy when they digest well. And most of their symptoms get worse when attacked by cold pathogens due to strong kidney water energy. Therefore, it is said that the pathological symptoms of the Shao Yin body type are mainly characterized by symptoms caused by the Stomach Cold and the Spleen/Kidney Yang Deficiency, which are poor digestion, incessant diarrhea, and streaming sweat, etc.

Regimen

Brown rice, potatoe, chicken, deer, lamb, goat, phasant, honey, pollack, anchovy, catfish, spinach, mugwart, green onion, ginger, pepper, mustard, black pepper, turmeric, scallions, apple, orange, mango, tomatoes, peach, dates, honey

Herbs

Ren Shen, Fu Zi, Rou Gui, Sha Ren, Gui Zhi, He Shou Wu, Bai Zhu, Cang Zhu, Dang Gui, Chuan Xiong, Ding Xiang, Mu Xiang, Gao Liang Jiang, Gan Jiang, Sheng Jiang, Huo Xiang, Xiang Fu, Ban Xia, Chen Pi, Qing Pi, Bai Shao, Bai Dou Kou, Rou Dou Kou, Huang Qi, Yi Zhi Ren, Wu Ling Zhi, Zi Su Ye, Yi Mu Cao, Shan Zha, Da Zao, Zhi Shi, Ba Dou, Yu Jin, Xi Xin, Du Zhong, Su He Xiang, Yin Chen, Su Mu, Nan Xing, San Qi, Gan Cao, Hou Pou, Ju Hong

Identification of Patterns and Formulas

The treasure of life for Shaoyins, the crucial factor for their health, is the warming Yang Qi. This is because they tend to get Excess Yin (Cold) and Deficient Yang (Heat) due to their strong Kidney water energy and weak Spleen energy, and most of their illnesses are caused by cold. Therefore, the basic mechanism of treatment for Shaoyins' illnesses is to boost up Yang Qi to expel the cold.

Exterior Syndrome

The treatment for Exterior Syndrome focuses on making the Kidney Yang Qi ascend. In Dr. Zhang's Shang Han Lun, Gui Zhi Tang is used for Exterior Deficiency (with sweating) and Ma Huang Tang is used for Exterior Excess (without sweating). However, in SCM Ma Huang (Ephedra) is considered as an herb for Tai Yin constitutions, but is not appropriate to use for deficient body types such as Shaoyins due to its ability to induce excessive perspiration. Dr. Lee used Huo Xiang, Zi Su Ye, Gui Zhi and Cong

Bai as releasing exterior herbs for Shaoyins. He adopted Gui Zhi Tang from Shang Han Lun, but modified with Spleen Qi tonic herbs, and Kidney Yang tonic herbs to make up for Shaoyins' constitutional weakness.

Formulas for Exterior Excess Syndrome

Chuan Xiong Gui Zhi Tang (川芎桂枝湯)
Chuanxiong Rhizoma and Cinnamon Twig Decoction

Sheng Jiang 12, Gui Zhi 8, Ban Xia 8, Bai Shao 4, Bai Zhu 4, Chen Pi 4, Zhi Gan Cao 4

This formula is for the early stage of Exterior Excess syndrome with chills and fever, no sweating, aversion to cold and wind, occipital headache, bodyaches, stiff neck, stuffy nose, and dry heaves.

Huo Xiang Zheng Qi San (藿香正氣散)
Agastache Powder to Rectify the Qi

Huo Xiang 6, Zi Su Ye 4, Cang Zhu 2, Bai Zhu 2, Ban Xia 2, Chen Pi 2, Qing Pi 2, Da Fu Pi 2, Gui Zhi 2, Gan Jiang 2, Yi Zhi Ren 2, Zhi Gan Cao 2

This formula can be used for the initial stage or the middle stage of Exterior Excess syndrome with chills and fever but no sweating, aversion to cold and wind, headache, bodyaches, and stiff neck. Besides this Tai Yang syndrome of 6 channel differentiation, it can be also used for Large Intestine Cold syndrome with Stomach pain and borborygmus, Yang Ming syndrome with unresolved exterior, and Tai Yin Syndrome with abdominal pain and diarrhea. This means it has a wide range of uses for both exterior and interior disorders.

Ba Wu Jun Zi Tang (八物君子湯)
Eight Noble Ingredients Decoction

Ren Shen 8, Huang Qi 4, Bai Zhu 4, Bai Shao 4, Dang Gui 4, Chuan Xiong 4, Chen Pi 4, Zhi Gan Cao 4, Sheng Jiang 4, Da Zao 3

This formula is for the early stage of Exterior Excess syndrome or Yang Ming Syndrome with dry mouth and constipation. Since it is a combination of the Four

Gentleman Decoction and the Four Substances Decoction, it can be used in almost any case where both the Qi and Blood is deficient. For the terminal stage of Exterior Excess syndrome, the dosage of Ren Shen can be increased up to 30-40g, and it becomes Du Shen Ba Wu Jun Zi Tang, which addresses Yang Ming Syndrome with tidal fever, manic speech, difficulty in breathing, and glassy eyes.

<u>Formulas for Exterior Deficiency Syndrome (Collapsed Yang in SCM)</u>

*Bu Zhong Yi Qi Tang(*補中益氣湯*)*
Tonify the Middle and Augment the Qi Decoction

Ren Shen 12, Huang Qi 12, Zhi Gan Cao 4, Bai Zhu 4, Dang Gui 4, Chen Pi 4, Sheng Jiang 4, Da Zao 3, Huo Xiang 1.2-2, Zi Su Ye 1.2-2,

This formula is modified from the famous Bu Zhong Yi Qi Tang of Dr. Li Dong-yuan. The original formula includes Chai Hu and Sheng Ma, which are for Shaoyangs and Taiyins respectively. By adding Huo Xiang and Zi Su Ye, this formula releases exterior wind cold, in addition to tonifying Qi of the middle burner and raising sunken Yang. It is for the early stages of Exterior Deficiency syndrome of the Shao Yin body type when there is tiredness and weakness, heat in the body, mental restlessness, spontaneous sweating, lethargy, and prolapse.

*Sheng Yang Yi Qi Tang (*升陽益氣湯*)*
Raise the Yang and Augment the Qi Decoction

Ren Shen 8, Gui Zhi 8, Huang Qi 8, Bai Shao 8, Bai He Shou Wu 4, Rou Gui 4, Dang Gui 4, Zhi Gan Cao 4, Sheng Jiang 4, Da Zao 3

This formula is for the early stage of Exterior Deficiency syndrome with chills and fever and spontaneous sweating. 4g of Fu Zi (Aconite) can be added to treat midstage Exterior Deficiency Syndrome, which manifests as Yang Ming syndrome with aversion to heat but no chills, spontaneous sweating, and frequent and clear urination. If the disease proceeds to the terminal stage of this syndrome of Collapsed Yang, body liquid deficiency occurs due to spontaneous sweating and frequent urination. The terminal stage symptoms include the Yang Ming syndrome with fever, profuse sweating, and dark yellow urine or urinary difficulty. In this case, Fu Zi needs to be increased to 8g.

Interior Syndrome

The Spleen Yang deficiency leads Shaoyins to be prone to digestive problems, which mainly include abdominal pain and diarrhea. As Interior Syndromes, Tai Yin Syndrome and Shao Yin Syndrome both have these two symptoms, but are different in that Shao Yin Syndrome also has thirst and an abnormal sensation of the mouth but Tai Yin Syndrome does not. Treatment for interior syndrome is focused on how to make the Excess Yin (cold) of Middle Jiao descend.

<u>Formulas for Tai Yin Syndrome</u>

Gui Zhi Ban Xia Sheng Jiang Tang (桂枝半夏生薑湯)
Cinnamon Twig, Pinellia, and Fresh Ginger Decoction

Sheng Jiang 12, Gui Zhi 8, Ban Xia 8, Bai Shao 4, Bai Zhu 4, Chen Pi 4, Zhi Gan Cao 4

This formula is modified from Gui Zhi Tang by adding Er Chen Tang and Bai Zhu and omitting Da Zao. It is used for Jiexiong (clumping in the chest or chest congestion) due to excess cold, Qi stagnation and phlegm fluids. The related symptoms are epigastric pain, nausea and vomiting, headache and bodyache.

Chi Bai He Wu Guan Zhong Tang (赤白何烏寬中湯)
Red and White Fo-Ti Root Decoction to Relieve the Middle

Bai He Shou Wu 4 Chi He Shou Wu 4 Gao Liang Jiang 4 Gan Jiang 4 Chen Pi 4 Qing Pi 4 Xiang Fu 4 Yi Zhi Ren 4 Da Zao 2

This formula is also used for Jiexiong Syndrome due to Excess Cold, but the difference is that this formula is also used for edema in addition to chest oppression. Edema in Shaoyins is usually accompanied by weak limbs, lethargy and dysuria.

Bai He Shou Wu Li Zhong Tang(白何首烏理中湯)
Regulate the Middle Decoction with White Fo-Ti

Bai He shou Wu 8, bai zhu 8, Bai Shao 8, Gui Zhi 4, Gan Jiang 4, Chen Pi 4, Zhi Gan Cao 4

This formula is indicated for stomach pain and diarrhea due to Spleen Yang deficiency. This is the modified Li Zhong Tang of Shang Han Lun and can be used for mild to moderate Tai Yin syndrome. By adding Fu Zi 4g, it becomes Bai He Shou Wu Fu Zi Li Zhong Tang, which is used in severe cases.

Xiang Sha Yang Wei Tang (香砂養胃湯)
Nourish the Stomach Decoction with Cyperus and Cardamon

Ren Shen 4, Bai Zhu 4, Bai Shao 4, Gan Cao 4, Ban Xia 4, Xiang Fu 4, Chen Pi 4, Gan Jiang 4, Shan Zha 4, Sha Ren 4, Bai Dou Kou 4, Sheng Jiang 4, Da Zao 2

This formula can be used for both exterior and interior syndrome. For Exterior Syndrome, this can resolve the Yang Ming symptoms of fullness and discomfort in the abdomen. It mainly treats the symptoms of Tai Yin, which are abdominal pain, epigastric distention, sweating, diarrhea and especially stomach pain and borborygmus due to Large Intestine Cold.

Huo Xiang Zheng Qi San (藿香正氣散)
Agastache Powder to Rectify the Qi

Huo Xiang 6, Zi Su Ye 4, Cang Zhu 2, Bai Zhu 2, Ban Xia 2, Chen Pi 2, Qing Pi 2, Da Fu Pi 2, Gui Zhi 2, Gan Jiang 2, Yi Zhi Ren 2, Zhi Gan Cao 2

This formula is also used for both Exterior and Interior disorders. Please refer to the explanation of this formula under Exterior Excess Syndrome.

Formulas for Shao Yin Syndrome

Guan Gui Fu Zi Li Zhong Tang (官桂附子理中湯)
Regulate the Middle Decoction with Cinnamon and Aconite

Ren Shen 12, Bai Zhu 8, Gan Jiang 8, Rou Gui 8, Bai Shao 4, Chen Pi 4, Zhi Gan Cao 4, Fu Zi 4-8

This formula is for Shao Yin Syndrome with abdominal pain, diarrhea, thirst, abnormal sensation of the mouth, bodyache, constant desire to sleep, and minute pulse. It is also modified from the Li Zhong Tang by increasing the dosage of Ren Shen and adding Bai Shao, Chen Pi, Rou Gui and Fu Zi to address Shao Yin Syndrome.

2. Shao Yang Constitution

<u>Points of differentiation</u>

Shaoyangs have a well-developed chest area which corresponds to the Spleen, but their hip area, which corresponds to the Kidneys, is relatively smaller and weaker. Some Shaoyang women with narrower hips may experience difficulty in conceiving due to weaker Kidney energy. Their face is usually smaller and oval with a thin and pointy jaw. Their eyes radiate a sharp and intense look. They tend to be outspoken and move quickly and do things in a hasty manner, which makes them look careless. Among celebrities, Bruce Lee has most physical traits of a typical Shao Yang constitution. Some Shaoyangs, especially in their later life, still can gain weight, but most Shaoyangs exude swift and agile impression. I better avoid mentioning too many celebrity names because physical aspects are not the only factor differentiating body types, but are only one of many, including psychological and pathophysiological aspects.

Shaoyangs are active, animated, and cheerful, and also good at exploring new experiences and pushing ahead with plans. However, they tend to be impatient in sticking to one project, and end up not being able to finish. They also love to take care of other's business rather than their own due to their tendency to extraversion. This can arouse anxiety and fearfulness, causing problems in family relationships, and if this goes to the extreme and they totally pursue achievements in the outside world, they can get more anxious and impulsive and do things on a whim without mature consideration.

Shaoyangs have a strong Spleen but weak kidneys. Therefore, their digestive systems are relatively strong, but their reproductive systems can be on the weaker side. It is said that Shaoyangs are healthy and sound if their bowel movements are regular. When they get constipated, they become vulnerable to pathogenic factors. Only 2-3 days of constipation still can cause Shaoyangs heaviness and stuffiness in their chest, which can lead to other serious illness. The congested feeling in the chest implies stagnation of excess yang (fire/heat) due to Kidney Yin (water/cold) deficiency. Prolonged imbalance of excess Yang and deficient Yin in Shao Yang constitution can later manifest as various types of Warm Febrile Diseases.

Regimen

Barley, Adzuki bean, green bean, pork, eggs, oyster, abalone, shrimp, crab, robster, carp, cucumber, cabbage, lettuce, eggplant, melon, strawberry, raspberry, banana

Herbs

Shu Di Huang, Sheng Di Huang, Rou Cong Rong, Gou Qi Zi, Fu Pen Zi, Shan Zhu Yu, Mu Dan Pi, Qiang Huo, Du Huo, Zhu Ling, Ze Xie, Chai Hu, Qian Hu, Jing Jie, Fang Feng, Huang Lian, Huang Bai, Gua Lou Ren, Niu Bang Zi, Di Gu Pi, Zhi Zi, Che Qian Zi, Jin Yin Hua, Ren Dong Teng, Ru Xiang, Mo Yao, Gan Sui, Da Ji, Ku Shen, Bo He, Zhu Sha, Xuan Shen, Lian Qiao, Mu Tong, Deng Xin Cao, Qu Mai, Shi Gao, Dong Kui Zi, Qing Hao, Hong Hua, Mang Xiao, Xia Ku Cao, Mu Zei, Zhi Mu, Fu Ling, Hai Jin Sha, Gui Ban

Identification of Patterns and Formulas

The treasure of life for Shaoyangs is the cooling Yin Qi. It is because they tend to get Excess Yang (Fire/Heat) and Deficient Yin (Water/Cold) due to their strong Spleen Yang energy and lack of Kidney Water energy. Therefore, the basic mechanism of treatment for Shaoyangs' illness is to nourish the deficient Yin thereby anchoring the floating Yang.

Exterior Syndrome

Dr. Lee said that, for Shaoyangs, interior heat attacking the stomach can cause constipation, and exterior cold affecting the spleen can cause diarrhea. So diarrhea or loose stool is one of the symptoms that indicates Exterior Syndrome in Shao Yang body types. Other symptoms include edema, coarse breathing, congestion in the chest, dysentery, alternating chills and fever, and distension in the chest and hypochondriac area. All these symptoms are due to congested Spleen Yin Qi not being able to descend.

13

Formulas for Wind Attack Syndrome

Shaoyang Wind Attack Syndrome manifests with fever, aversion to cold, floating and tight pulse, bodyaches, lack of perspiration, and restlessness. Other symptoms include bitter taste in the mouth, dry throat, dizziness, tinnitus, fullness and distension in the chest and hypochondrium, alternating chills and fever, and nausea.

Jing Fang Bai Du San (荊防敗毒散)
Detoxify Pathogens Powder with Schizonepata and Siler

Qiang Huo 4 Du Huo 4 Chai Hu 4 Qian Hu 4 Jing Jie 4 Fang Feng 4 Chi Fu Ling 4 Sheng Di Huang 4 Di Gu Pi 4 Che Qian Zi 4

This formula is mainly for the Exerior Excess of Wind Cold, with symptoms such as headache, bodyache, neck stiffness, and chills and fever. Secondarily, it can also be used for Shao Yang disorder with alternating chills and fever, bitter taste in the mouth, dry mouth, vertigo and hypochondriac fullness/distention. Belching and sudden vomiting in Shaoyangs can also be addressed with this formula.

Jing Fang Dao Chi San (荊防導赤散)
Guide Out the Red with Schizonepata and Siler Powder

Sheng Di Huang 12, Che Qian Zi 8, Xuan Shen 6, Gua Lou Ren 6, Qian Hu 4, Qiang Huo 4, Du Huo 4, Jing Jie 4, Fang Feng 4

Indications of this formula are headache, irritability, thirst, delirium, and severe chest congestion with shoulder pain and neck stiffness. Secondary symptoms are nausea, vomiting, fullness in the epigastrium, and shortness of breath. All of these are the manifestations of Jiexiong syndrome.

Jing Fang Xie Bai San(荊防瀉白散)
Sedate the White with Schizonepata and Sileris Powder

Sheng Di Huang 12, Fu Ling 8, Ze Xie 8, Shi Gao 4, Zhi Mu 4, Qiang Huo 4, Du Huo 4, Jing Jie 4, Fang Feng 4

This treats exterior disorder showing more heat signs and symptoms such as irritability, restlessness in the hands and feet, flu with fever, headache, and ear infection. It can be applied to disorders of Hyperactivity due to heat such as ADHD, tics, hypertension, anxiety, and insomnia.

Formulas for Collapsed Yin Syndrome (Mang Yin 亡陰)

Mang Yin is a unique disorder for Shaoyangs in SCM, which is mainly characterized by diarrhea. The clinical manifestations include Cholera, acute/chronic colitis, Irritable Bowel Syndrome, and functional dyspepsia. Chronic diarrhea in Shaoyangs causes dehydration with electrolyte imbalance and needs to tonify Yin.

Jing Fang Di Huang Tang (荊防地黃湯)
Rehmannia with Schizonepata and Sileris Decoction

Shu Di Huang 8, Shan Zhu Yu 8, Fu Ling 8, Ze Xie 8, Che Qian Zi 4, Qiang Huo 4, Du Huo 4, Jing Jie 4, Fang Feng 4

The indication for this formula is headache, abdominal pain, abdominal bloating, and diarrhea. It is commonly used for Collapse Yin Syndrome with coldness for Shaoyangs.

Hua Shi Ku Shen Tang (滑石苦蔘湯)
Talcum and Sophora Decoction

Ze Xie 8, Fu Ling 8, Hua Shi 8, Ku Shen 8, Huang Lian 4, Huang Bai 4, Qiang Huo 4, Du Huo 4, Jing Jie 4, Fang Feng 4

This formula treats Yin Collapse Syndrome with coldness. The signs and symptoms include chest and abdominal pain, stomach cramps, diarrhea, and coldness in the body.

Zhu Ling Che Qian Zi Tang (猪笭車前子湯)
Polyporus and Plantain Decoction

Ze Xie 8, Fu Ling 8, Zhu Ling 6, Che Qian Zi 6, Zhi Mu 4, Shi Gao 4, Qiang Huo 4, Du Huo 4, Jing Jie 4, Fang Feng 4,

The indication for this formula is headache, abdominal pain, diarrhea, fever, and difficulty urinating. It is used for Collapsed Yin Syndrome with heat signs and symptoms.

Jing Fang Xie Bai San (荊防瀉白散)
Sedate the White with Schizonepata and Sileris Powder

Sheng Di Huang 12, Fu Ling 8, Ze Xie 8, Shi Gao 4, Zhi Mu 4, Qiang Huo 4, Du Huo 4, Jing Jie 4, Fang Feng 4

This can be used for Collapsed Yin syndrome with Heat. It is explained further under Wind Attack Syndrome.

Interior Syndrome

As mentioned in Exterior Syndrome, Shaoyangs get constipated when the Stomach is attacked by interior heat and get diarrhea when the Spleen is attacked by exterior cold. Therefore, hard stool due to heat can cause various symptoms of Interior Syndrome in the Shao Yang Body type. After the Stomach is attacked by heat, if Shaoyangs have constipation and no bowel movement for about 3 days, the body can perspire, depleting the clear Yang Qi. When the clear Yang Qi cannot rise to the head and empty fire stagnates in the head and limbs instead, various symptoms can occur including stroke, hematemesis, vomiting, abdominal pain, food stagnation, and fullness and distension. All these symptoms are due to the clear Kidney Yang Qi not being able to ascend.

Formulas for Excess Yang Syndrome

Liang Ge San Huo Tang (凉膈散火)
Cool the Diaphragm and Disperse the Fire Decoction

Sheng Di Huang 8 Ren Dong Teng 8 Lian Qiao 8 Zhi Zi 4 Bo He 4 Zhi Mu 4 Shi Gao 4 Fang Feng 4 Jing Jie 4

This formula is used for polydipsia, restlessness and stuffiness in the chest, sore throat, swelling lips, tongue ulcers, and abnormal sweating.

Ren Dong Teng Di Gu Pi Tang (忍冬藤地骨皮湯)
Honeysuckle Stem and Lycium Bark Decoction

Ren Dong Teng 16, Shan Zhu Yu 8, Di Gu Pi 8, Huang Lian 8, Huang Bai 8, Xuan Shen 4, Ku Shen 4, Sheng Di Huang 4, Zhi Mu 4, Zhi Zi 4, Gou Qi Zi 4, Fu Pen Zi 4, Jing Jie 4, Fang Feng 4, Jin Yin Hua 4

This formula is used for polyphagia with heat accumulation in the Middle Jiao.

Di Huang Bai Hu Tang (地黃白虎湯)
White Tiger with Rehmannia Decoction

Shi Gao 20-40, Sheng Di Huang 16, Zhi Mu 8, Fang Feng 4, Du Huo 4

When Shaoyangs cannot pass stools more than once a day, this formula needs to be administered to clear interior heat. Prolonged constipation can lead to other serious heat conditions such as irritability, delirious utterances, stiff tongue, and manic behavior with screaming.

Formulas for Deficient Yin Syndrome

Shu Di Huang Ku Shen Tang (熟地黃苦蔘湯)
Rehmannia with Pubescent Angelica Decoction

Shu Di Huang 16, Shan Zhu Yu 8, Fu Ling 6, Ze Xie 6, Huang Bai 4, Ku Shen 4, Zhi Mu 4

This treats polyuria, placenta not descending, frequent and difficult urination, and soreness and pain in joints. All of these are due to latent Heat in the lower burner.

Du Huo Di Huang Tang (獨活地黃湯)
Rehmannia with Pubescent Angelica Decoction

Shu Di Huang 16, Shan Zhu Yu 8, Fu Ling 6, Ze Xie 6, Mu Dan Pi 4, Fang Feng 4, Du Huo 4

The indications for this formula are indigestion, bloating, Deficient Heat, stroke, vomiting, early stage of Bell's Palsy, low back pain, knee pain, and infertility.

Shi Er Wei Di Huang Tang (十二味地黃湯)
Twelve Ingredients with Rehmannia Decoction

Shu Di Huang 16, Shan Zhu Yu 8, Fu Ling 6, Ze Xie 6, Mu Dan Pi 4, Di Gu Pi 4, Xuan Shen 4, Gou Qi Zi 4, Fu Pen Zi 4, Che Qian Zi 4, Jing Jie 4, Fang Feng 4

This formula is used for hematemesis, Deficient Heat, hernia, and epilepsy.

3. Tai Yin Constitution

Points of differentiation

Taiyins have strong Liver and weak Lungs. The Liver's function is to store blood and the Liver Qi is easily stagnated. Thus Taiyins naturally accumulate Qi and blood easily rather than eliminating it, which causes them to gain weight especially around the waist area that corresponds to the Liver. Their face is usually round or square, their skin is relatively thick, and they usually sweat easily. The famous actress Conchata Ferrell, who played Berta the housekeeper for the sitcom *Two and a Half Men,* is a classic example of Tai Yin body type.

As for personality, Taiyins are mostly calm, laidback, patient, persistent, and pragmatic. They have a great sense of responsibility, and eventually accomplish their goals. They tend to prefer staying still and are unwilling to move around. This causes them to only take care of their own business and family and not consider the outside world. If this goes to the extreme, it can arouse fear in their mind and they can become more mistrustful, closed minded, and cowardly. As their organ imbalance causes a natural accumulation of substances rather than an elimination, when it comes to the imbalance of their life, they can become greedy and possessive, not sharing anything but constantly trying to acquire more.

Their physical condition is good when they sweat freely. If there is no sweat with firmer skin and closed pores, it indicates an unhealthy state for Taiyins and can lead to a more serious illness. The accumulated waste in their body can be somewhat released with sweating during exercise. While Shaoyins get tired after sweating, Taiyins become refreshed and revitalized after sweating.

The overaccumulation of substances combined with the slow metabolism in Taiyin can cause heat congestion that leads to Dryness in the Lungs and Heat in the Liver. More often than not Taiyin can get constipated easily due to a high appetite and slow metabolism. However, diarrhea or dysentery in this constitution can be counted as a more serious condition. Overall we can say that Taiyins are healthy when they are able to release their accumulated substances through sweat, urination and bowel movement. The malfunction of these three such as no sweating, urinary difficulty and constipation can generate Dry Heat Syndrome, which is the main characteristic of the pathological syndrome of Tai Yin body type.

Regimen

wheat, beans, pearl barley, tofu, yam, almond, beef, milk, cod, eel, seaweeds, radish, carrot, bellflower root, lotus root, mushrooms, chestnut, bean sprout, chestnut, pine nut, walnut, gingko, pear, apricot, plum, prune

Herbs

Lu Rong, Long Yan Rou, Niu Huang, Mai Men Dong, Tian Men Dong, Bai Zi Ren, Lian Zi, Yi Yi Ren, Lai Fu Zi, Jie Geng, Sheng Ma, Huang Qin, Bai Zhi, Yuan Zhi, Shi Chang Pu, Bai Guo, Da Huang, Ma Zi Ren, Kuan Dong Hua, Suan Zao Ren, Gao Ben, Shan Yao, Bei Mu, Fu Ping, She Gan, Wu Mei, Xing Ren, Sang Bai Pi, Wu Wei Zi, Shi Jun Zi, Xu Duan, Pu Gong Ying, Wei Ling Xian, Pu Huang, She Chuang Zi, Sha Shen, Ze Lan, Quan Xie[14], Chuan Shan Jia[15], Sang Ji Sheng, Tu Fu Ling, Tian Ma, Hu Gu

Identification of Patterns and Formulas

The treasure of life for Taiyins is dispersing Qi. It is because they tend to absorb and accumulate substances in the body due to their strong Liver energy and weak Lung energy. Therefore, the basic mechanism of treatment for Taiyins is to disperse and eliminate overaccumulated Qi and Body fluids.

---

[14] scorpion

[15] pangolin

Exterior Syndrome

When Taiyins are attacked by exterior cold, the cold-dampness tends to be accumulated in the epigastrium area. So the Exterior Syndrome is differentiated based on whether the symptoms of food stagnation exist, in addition to any cold/flu symptoms.

The Formulas for Exterior Cold

*Ma Huang Fa Biao Tang (*麻黃發表湯*)*
Ephedra Decoction to Release Exterior

Jie Geng 12, Ma Huang 6, Mai Men Dong 4, Huang Qin 4, Xing Ren 4

For a light condition of the Cold Jue (寒厥) syndrome of Tai Yang disorder. This treats Wind-Cold condition with bodyache, lumbago, arthralgia, cough or wheezing, feverish headache, and chills without sweating.

*Han Duo Re Shao Tang (*寒多熱少湯*)*
Greater Cold and Lesser Heat Decoction

Yi Yi Ren 12, Gan Li 12 (dried chest nut), Lai fu zi 8, Huang Qin 4, Mai Men Dong 4, Xing Ren 4, Jie Geng 4, Ma Huang 4

For severe conditions of the Cold Jue syndrome of Tai Yang disorder. It treats Cold Jue on the fourth or fifth day without sweating. As Dr. Zhang said, there must be a fever on the fourth to fifth day of Jue. Extreme Jue will lead to a high fever. When Jue is slight, the fever will also be slight. For febrile disease caused by cold, Jue lasts for 4 days, followed by fever for 3 days. Having more days of fever than Jue foretells a recovery. Dr. Lee said Jue in this case means the sensation of chills without fever, but it does not mean cold limbs.

The Formulas for Cold Syndrome in the epigastrium

*Tai Yin Tiao Wei Tang*太陰調胃湯
Decoction for Taiyins to Regulate the Stomach

Yi Yi Ren 12, Gan Li 12, Lai Fu Zi 8, Wu Wei Zi 4, Mai Men Dong 4, Shi Chang Pu 4, Jie Geng 4, Ma Huang 4

For a light condition of Cold syndrome in the Epigastrium. This treats jaundice, headache, bodyache, wind cold symptoms without sweating, indigestion with discomfort and fullness, and weakness of legs.

Tiao Wei Cheng Qing Tang(調胃升清湯)
Regulate the Stomach and Raise the Clear Decoction

Yi Yi Ren 12, Gan Li 12, Lai Fu Zi 6, Ma Huang 4, Jie Geng 4, Mai Men Dong 4, Wu Wei Zi 4, Shi Chang Pu 4, Yuan Zhi 4, Tian Men Dong 4, Suan Zao Ren 4, Long Yan Rou 4

For severe Cold syndrome in the Epigastrium. The indications for this formula are distention and fullness after meals, weak legs, and constant hunger.

Interior Syndrome

When Qi and Body fluids are overaccumulated, Liver heat is generated in Tai Yin body types due to strong Liver energy. This Liver heat causes dryness in the Lungs, and eventually the dry heat condition leads to exhaustion of both Yin and Blood in the body.

<u>The Formulas for Dry Heat Syndrome</u>

Ge Gen Jie Ji Tang (葛根解肌湯)
Release the Muscle Layer Decoction with Kudzu

Ge Gen 12, Huang Qin 6, Gao Ben 6, Jie Geng 4, Sheng Ma 4, Bai Zhi 4

For a light condition of Dry Heat Syndrome. The indications of this formula are slight chills and fever, orbital and eye pain, dry nasal cavity, insomnia of Yang Ming disorder. It can treat Yangdu (陽毒) symptoms like silky patterns of red spots on the face, sore throat, hemoptysis with pus. This formula is also for severe thirst and delirious speech, gastric ulcer or gastritis with foul belching and sour regurgitation, and headaches with flushing and fever. The original text also indicates that it can be used for Cold Jue without sweating for five days.

Angie Kim, Ph.D., L.Ac.

Re Duo Han Shao Tang (熱多寒少湯)
Greater Heat and Lesser Cold Decoction

Ge Gen 16, Huang Qin 8, Gao Ben 8, Lai Fu Zi 4, Jie Geng 4, Sheng Ma 4, Bai Zhi 4

For severe conditions of Dry Heat Syndrome. The indication of this formula is lethargy, spermatorrhea, and the disease manifesting burnt black colored fingers and gangrenous changes. It can also be used for Diabetes with thirst, constipation, excess water consumption, and a large volume of urine.

The Formuals for Yin Blood Exhaustion Syndrome

Lu Rong Da Bu Tang (鹿茸大補湯)
Deer Antler Decoction for Great Tonification

Lu Rong 8-16, Mai Men Dong 6, Yi Yi Ren 6, Shan Yao 4, Tian Men Dong 4, Wu Wei Zi 4, Xing Ren 4, Ma Huang 4

For the exterior symptoms of Yin Blood Exhaustion Syndrome. This can be used for deficient and weak conditions with various external cold symptoms. The deficient condition manifests as deafness, visual difficulty, weakness in the legs, lower back pain, and spermatorrhea.

Gong Chen He Yuan Dan (拱辰黑元丹)
Modified Gong Chen Dan for Black Vitality

Lu Rong 16-24, Shan Yao 16, Tian Men Dong 16, Qi Cao 4-8

For interior symptoms of Yin Blood Exhaustion Syndrome. This can be used for deficient and weak Taiyins only with interior symptoms such as deafness, visual difficulty, weakness in the legs, lower back pain,and spermatorrhea.

4. Tai Yang Constitution

Points of differentiation

Tai Yang constitution, known as the greater Yang compared to the lesser Yang (Shao Yang), has more noticeable development in upper body (yang) and a less developed lower body (yin). Therefore, their Pectoralis Major is well developed, and the head and neck area is also bigger than on other body types. The lower portion from the waist down, which corresponds to the Liver, is rather weak. Their standing posture looks unstable due to their small buttocks and weak legs. Their facial characteristics are clearly defined with sharp and piercing eyes creating an intense and aggressive look. Taiyangs are the rarest body type: imagine the character Hercules in the Walt Disney animated film.

Taiyangs make friends easily because they are very social and have good communication skills. They are extremely creative, highly intelligent and naturally inquisitive. Due to their excessive Yang energy, they always want to move forward and are typically hotheaded and reckless. Yang is masculine energy, and when this energy goes to the extreme, Taiyangs can be cocky, self-indulgent, self-righteous, and easily fall into heroism.

Taiyangs possess strong lungs and a weak liver. As opposed to Taiyins, they naturally disperse Qi and eliminate substances easily rather than accumulating them. Therefore, most of their issues stem from too much dispersal of Yang energy upward and too little storage of body substances. Taiyangs are healthy if they urinate well, because urination indicates that the energy is moving downward within the body. If their energy goes upward too much, it can cause excessive foamy saliva, dysphagia, and vomiting, which needs to be addressed immediately. Excess in the upper body leads to deficiency in the lower body. The associated symptoms are lower back pain, weakness in the lower body, and difficulty walking. If symptoms gets more serious, they may also experience weight loss and severe fatigue, not even wanting to talk or move.

Regimen

buckwheat, clam, oyster, abalone, crab, squid, octopus, pine leaf, green leafy vegetables, grapes, persimmon, cherry, pine flower, Siberian gooseberry

Herbs

Lu Gen, Mu Gua, Ying Tao Rou[16], Song Jie[17], Song Hua[18], Wu Jia Pi, Pu Tao Gen[19], Mi Hou Tao[20]

Identification of Patterns and Formulas

The treasure of life for Taiyangs is storing Qi. It is because they tend to disperse and eliminate substances easily due to their strong Lung energy and weak Liver energy. Therefore, the essential point to treat Taiyangs' symptoms is to restore Qi and Body fluids.

Exterior Syndrome

As reviewed during the discussion of the theory of visceral groups in SCM, the constituents of the liver group are the liver, small intestine, nose, lumbar region and muscles. An attack by an exterior pathogen in this body type can damage the exterior Qi of the lumbar region, which causes weakness in the lower body. This is the Jieyi (解㑊) Syndrome of Taiyangs. They are perfectly healthy in the upper body, but fatigued in the lower body, so they are unable to walk. However, the leg is not swollen nor paralyzed nor painful, and neither too cold nor too hot.

---

[16] cherry
[17] knotty pine wood
[18] pine flower
[19] grape root
[20] Siberian gooseberry

Formula for Jieyi (解㑊)

Wu Jia Pi Zhuang Ji Tang (五加皮壯脊湯)
Strengthen the Spine Decoction with Acanthopanax

Wu Jia Pi 16 Mu Gua 8 Qing Song Jie 8 Pu Tao Gen 4 Lu Gen 4 Ying Tao Rou 4 Qiao Mai Mi 4

This formula strengthens the spine, sinews, and muscles, and treats Jieyi (解㑊) syndrome, which is the exterior disorder of Taiyangs.

Interior Syndrome

As the Small Intestine is a part of the Liver Group, when anger bursts out of them, not only the Liver is weakened but also the Small Intestine gets damaged. This manifests as Dysphasia(Yege) or vomiting(Fanwei). Symptoms can occur when the Small Intestine of Taiyangs cannot absorb Qi and Body Fluids, and the Qi in the epigastrium is dispersed excessively.

Formula for Yege(噎膈) or Fanwei(反胃)

Mi Hou Teng Zhi Chang Tang (獼猴籐植腸湯)
Plant the Intestine Decoction with Actinidia

Mi Hou Tao 16, Mu Gua 8, Pu Tao Gen 8, Lu Gen 4, Ying Tao Rou 4, Wu Jia Pi 4, Song Hua 4, Chu Tou Tang(bran) 4

This formula is for internal disorders of Taiyangs, mainly for Dysphasia(Yege) or vomiting(Fanwei). It can be used for digestive disorders such as loose stool, indigestion, and stuffiness in the epigastic region, and also for neurotic disorders such as restlessness, anxiety, headache, and the symptoms of blood rushing to the head.

5. Later Studies

There have been efforts to develop SCM from the overall approach of evidence based medicine (EBM), integrating both western allopathic and holistic traditional medicine. The studies vary from investigations into diagnostic methods to improve accuracy of diagnosis to explorations of the development of systems of constitution.

Among those, Eight Constitutional Medicine(ECM)[21] by Dr. Kuon Dowon is the most creative outcome in that he revealed the strengths and weaknesses of all ten organs along with the activity of sympathetic and parasympathetic nerve systems in each of the eight different body types and applied his theory to acupuncture treatments.

"The human body consists of 10 organs altogether: five solid organs and five hollow organs. From the point of conception, these organs develop and fall into an order of strong and weak, and the groupings of these orders that are distinguishable from each other total eight. This is the fundamental, underlying principle of the eight constitutions, with the strengths and weakness of the organs being directly related to their size.

That said, the condition in which the liver is the largest organ with the nine remaining organs ordered according to strength and weakness is called Hepatonia, while the condition where the pancreas is largest is called Pancretonia, that with the stomach is the largest Gastrotonia, that with the lungs as the largest Pulmotonia, that with the colon as the largest Colonotonia, that with the kidneys as largest Renotonia, and that with the bladder as the largest Vesicotonia.

---

[21] The eight constitutions are;
  Renotonia (water yang): Kidney > Lung > Liver >Heart > Pancreas
  Vesicotonia(water yin): Urinary Bladder > Gall Bladder > Small Intestine > Large Intestine> Stomach
  Hepatonia (wood yang): Liver > Kidney > Heart > Pancreas > Lung
  Cholecystonia (wood yin): Gall Bladder > Small Intestine >Stomach> Urinary Bladder > Large Intestine
  Pulmotonia(metal yang): Lung > Pancreas > Heart > Kidney > Liver
  Colonotonia(metal yin): Large Intestine>Urinary Bladder>Stomach>Small Intestine> Gall Bladder
  Pancreotonia (earth yang): Pancreas > Heart > Liver > Lung > Kidney
  Gastrotonia (earth yin): Stomach > Large Intestine >Small Intestine > Gall Bladder > Urinary Bladder
  - From *heavenly regimen* by CMC research group (Korean version)

Among these eight constitutions, there are four in which the sympathetic nervous system is always in a tense state. The grouping of these is called sympathicotonia, and includes Pulmotonia, Colonotonia, Renotonia, and Vesicotonia. The other grouping is called Vagotonia, in which the parasympathetic nervous system is always in a tense state, and includes Hepatonia, Cholecystonia, Pancreotonia, and Gastrotonia. One of the characteristics of those with a constitution grouped under Vagotonia is that beneficial for them drink caffeinated coffe or other caffeinated drinks. Those who fall under the category of Sympathicotonia should not drink caffeinated coffee.

Recently, the results of a comparative examination of the degree of activity of Amylase in the saliva of people from each of eight constitutions at Dong-A University in Busan (South Korea) revealed that Amylase was high in the four Sympathicotonia constitutions, while it was low in the four Vagotonia constitution."

From *Eight Constitutional Medicine: An overview* by Dr. Kuon Dowon

Although this book mainly discusses herbs and formulas, its consideration of the relative strength of every organ for each constitution is still valuable when customizing the formulas precisely. And also it can be a clue to determine body type and to check how people respond to caffeine in their daily lives. Some can get jittery and insomniac after drinking coffee, while others only get more energetic or even suffer from somnolence.

In ECM, the administration of vitamin supplements and medications per each body type has been studied in addition to food regimens. For example, vitamin B supplement is the most beneficial for Shaoyins, vitamin E supplement is for Shaoyangs, and vitamin D supplement for Taiyins. And taking a tablet of baby Aspirin everyday can prevent many diseases in the body type of Hepatonia.

Further studies are needed on the efficacy of western medicines in relation to each body type. Due to Americans' higher use of western medical drugs, this study would also play a role in discerning body types as a diagnostic method.

Chapter 2

Japanese Studies

Japanese traditional medicine is known as Kampo medicine. It means 'Chinese style medicine', and it is primarily concerned with the study of herbs. Since the 7th century, when traditional Chinese medicine was introduced by way of Korea, the Japanese have created their own unique system of diagnosis and therapy.

1. Todo Yoshimasu

Dr. Todo Yoshimasu (1702–1773) is one of the most influential figures in Kampo herbal medicine history.

The differences between Japanese Kampo medicine and the traditional forms of medicine in China and Korea are primarily due to the changes that were implemented by Dr. Todo Yoshimasu, who effectively constructed the basis for modern medicine in Japan. He questioned medical theories based on yin yang five phase metaphysics, and he put together a unique system of medicine based on the *Shang Han Lun* and the *Jin Gui Yao Lue*. He collected each of the formulas described in the chapters on the 220 formulas in the Shang Han Lun and Jin Gui Yao Lue, added his own opinions and published the resulting manuscript under the title *Ruijuho*類聚方 to present the standards for 'Koho' or traditional methods of treating patients. In addition, he collected information on the indications for various herbs and published a manuscript called *Yakucho*藥徵, in which he described analogous pharmacologic effects for the individual herbs contained in those formulas.[22]

---

[22] Hiromichi Yasui, <Medical History in Japan>, The Journal of Kampo, Japan Institute of TCM Research, 2007

There are some important points which can be found in his or his disciples' books.

First, all diseases are caused by a single poison. Therefore, the treatment should be geared toward removing the toxin of the disease from the body by attacking it with a medicine, which is also a poison itself. The location of toxin is confirmed by 'fukushin' (abdominal diagnosis), and the patient is treated with a formula that accurately targets the patient's symptoms. The toxin of disease can generate all the symptoms, but not all symptoms can inform the location of the toxin. So the symptom that informs the location of the toxin is very important and is called as the main indication.[23]

Second, there is no medicine used to replenish vital energy or essence since medicine is also a poison and it only attacks the toxin. This is why he criticized the conventional pharmacology based on the *Shen Nong Ben Cao Jing*, a Chinese book on agriculture and medicinal plants, and insisted that the Shang Han Lun should be used instead. In other words, he believed that, in the medical arts, only a method of attack existed, a method of replenishment did not. When the toxin is attacked by medicine, there occurs Ming Xuan 暝眩, a medical reaction as a healing sign.

The third treatment principle is 'relating symptoms to medicine,' based on a complete understanding of the indication of formula, not based on etiology and pathogenesis nor by the name of disease. Dr. Todo emphasized grasping the indication of the formula and tried to ignore the contexts which were related to Shang Han Lun. He said he used six channel differentiation only as a way of classification, that the more important thing was the symptom complex.

Fourth, never speak of what you cannot see with your eyes. Because he was unable to see within the body, he refused to say anything about that. Since he could not analyze the mechanism of etiologic pathogenesis, he refused to accept the theories of traditional medicine.[24] He also held that the medical explanation based on the yin yang five element theory and visceral concept does not help at all in treating diseases.

---

[23] Lee Junghuan and Jung Changhyun, <Yakucho of Todo Yoshimasu>, Chung Hong, 2006 (Korean version)

[24] Hiromichi Yasui, <Medical History in Japan>, The Journal of Kampo, Japan Institute of TCM Research, 2007

The new Meji government, which took control of Japan in 1868, adopted a German medical model, and Kampo medicine ceased to be in the mainstream of Japanese medical practice. However, Kampo continued to be popular among the common people, and even experienced a certain level of revival. Since that process of revival was based on Yoshimasu's theories, modern Kampo medicine in Japan closely resembles his teachings. Clearly Yoshimasu's tradition continues to live in Japan today.[25]

2. Yakucho(藥徵)

Dr. Todo Yoshimasu wrote the book *Yakucho* about the efficacy of herbs that were used in the *Shang Han Lun* and *Jin Gui Yao Lue*. This is the last book written by him and was completed in 1771, two years before he passed away. However, it was not published while he was alive since he wanted further review and revision. It was in 1785, 12 years after his death, that this book was finally published by his disciples.

In the author's preface, he stated how he found out the indication of each herb. First, he sorted out the sentences from *Shang Han Lun* and *Jin Gui Yao Lue* that might prove the indications of herbs. Second, if he couldn't find the proof from those two books, he collected formulas from other books that include the same herbs and compared each other. And last, he figured out which information was right or wrong based on old teachings and added his contemplations.

Yakucho can be translated as signs and symptoms of herbs. The main indications of herbs from *Yakucho*[26] are as follow.

Shi Gao

Shi Gao mainly treats thirst. Secondarily it treats delirious speech, irritability and agitation, and generalized heat.

The indications above are deduced from the formulas of Bai Hu Tang, Bai Hu Jia Ren Shen Tang, and Bai Hu Jia Gui Zhi Tang.

---

[25] Ibid

[26] Dr. Todo's Yakucho is translated into Korean by Lee Junghuan and Jung Changhyun, in the book, <Yakucho of Todo Yoshimasu>, Chung Hong, 2006

Hua Shi

Hua Shi mainly treats inhibited urination. Secondarily treats thirst.

These indications are based on the formula of Zhu Ling Tang.

Mang Xiao

Mang Xiao softens hardness. Therefore, it can treat focal distention and hardness below the heart, congested lesser abdomen, obstruction in the chest (jie xiong), dry stool, and hard stool. Secondarily can treat undigested food, fullness in the abdomen, and hardness and abscess in the lesser abdomen.

Gan Cao

Gan Cao mainly treats urgency. Therefore it can treat abdominal urgency, urgent pain, and urgent cramps. Secondarily it can treat various urgent toxins related to coldness (jue), irritability and agitation, and surging counterflow.

In Shang Han Lun, Dr. Zhang said, "when in lesser yin disease that has lasted for two or three days, there is sore throat, one can give Gan Cao Tang. If the person does not recover, give Jie Geng Tang"[27] The indication of Gan Cao can be understood based on this as well.

Huang Qi

Huang Qi treats water in the skin. Therefore, it can treat yellow sweat,[28] nightsweat, and skin discharge. Also, secondarily it treats swelling and numbness.

On the discusuion of Huang Qi Gui Zhi Wu Wu Tang, Dr. Zhang stated that there is numbness in the body. After comparing different formulas addressing numbness,

---

[27] Craig Mitchelle, Feng Ye, Nigel Wiseman, <Shang Han Lun>, Paradigm Publications

[28] Refers to perspiration of yellow colored sweat which often even stains the patient's clothings. 'Huang Han' in Pin Yin.
Philippe Sionneau &Lu Gang , <The treatment of Disease in TCM>, Blue Poppy Press, 2000

Dr. Todo realized that Dr. Zhang used herbs to treat water when treating numbness. He concluded that numbness is the disease of water.

Ren Shen

Ren Shen mainly treats focal distention, hardness, vertical prolonged congestion below the heart. Secondarily it treats anorexia, vomiting, frequent expectoration of saliva, heart pain, abdominal pain, irritability and palpitation.

Dr. Todo assumed that Ren Shen, Huang Lian and Fu Ling have similar functions. Ren Shen treats palpitation with distention and hardness below the heart, Huang Lian treats palpitation with irritability, and Fu Ling treats the palpitation with muscle twitches.

Jie Geng

Jie Geng treats turbid sputum, swelling and abscess. Secondarily it can also treat sore throat.

This indication is based on Jie Geng Tang and San Wu Bai San. Pai Nong Tang, which include Jie Geng as the king herb, did not have the indication of Jie Geng, but the name of the formula shows the Jie Geng's function of treating abcess because it means 'a formula releasing abscess'.

Zhu

There are Bai Zhu and Cang Zhu. Both have the same indication, but Cang Zhu has stronger efficacy, as Dr. Todo indicated. Since Dr. Todo didn't believe in Tonic herbs, Cang Zhu is more appropriate.

Zhu treats water. Therefore it can treat frequent urination and inhibited urination. Secondarily, it also treats burning bodyaches, phlegm-fluids, spermatorrhea, veiling dizziness, diarrhea, and frequent expectoration of saliva.

Bai Tou Weng

Bai Tou Weng treats heat diarrhea with rectal heaviness, which means loose stool accompanied by a feeling of heat and pressure in the anus.[29]

This indication is based on Bai Tou Weng Tang and Bai Tou Weng Jia Gan Cao E Jiao Tang.

Huang Lian

Huang Lian mainly treats irritability and palpitation. Secondarily treats focal distention below the heart, vomiting, diarrhea, and pain in the abdomen.

Huang Qin

Huang Qin treats focal distention below the heart. Scondarily, it also treats fullness in the chest and hypochondrium, vomiting and diarrhea.

Chai Hu

Chai Hu treats fullness and discomfort in the chest and hypochondrium. Secondarily treats alternating chills and fever, pain in the abdomen, distention and hardness in the hypochondrium.

Bei Mu

Bei Mu mainly treats congested phegm-fluids in the chest and diaphragm.

This indication is from Jie Geng Bai San.

---

[29] Craig Mitchelle, Feng Ye, Nigel Wiseman, <Shang Han Lun>, Paradigm Publications

Xie Xin

Xie Xin mainly treats abiding fluids and water. Therefore, it treats cough due to water in the epigastrium, fullness, upward conterflow, and pain in the hypochondrium.

Shao Yao

Shao Yao mainly treats hypertonicity of muscles. Secondarily treats abdominal pain, headaches, bodyaches, numbness, fullness in the abdomen, cough, diarrhea, and swelling with abscess.

Based on the formulas of Gui Zhi Jia Shao Yao Tang, Xiao Jian Zhong Tang and Gui Zhi Jia Da Huang Tang, Dr. Todo identified the nature of pain that Shao Yao treats, which is cramping and contracting due to hypertonicity of the muscles.

Yin Chen Hao

Yin Chen Hao mainly treats Jaundice.

When there is jaundice with inhibited urination and thirst, Yin Chen Wu Ling San is used. When there is jaundice with constipation, Yin Chen Hao Tang is used.

Ma Huang

Ma Huang mainly treats panting, cough, and Water qi[30]. Secondarily treats aversion to wind, aversion to cold, no sweating, generalized pain, joint pain, generalized yellow discoloration and swelling.

---

[30] Pathological excesses of water in the body. This term can refer to the water swelling provoked by it or other signs related to collected water. The main cause is impairment of movement and transformation of water.
- Craig Mitchelle, Feng Ye, Nigel Wiseman, <Shang Han Lun>, Paradigm Publications

Di Huang

Di Huang mainly treats inhibited urination and symptoms related to blood.

Ting Li

Ting Li mainly treats disorders of Water.

Da Huang

Da Huang mainly expel toxins.Therefore, it can treats fullness in the chest and abdomen, abdominal pain, constipation, and inhibited urination. Secondarily treats jaundice, blood stagnation, swelling and abscess.

Fu Zi

Fu Zi mainly expels water. Therefore it can treat chills, bodyaches, pain in the joints and limbs, heaviness, numbness, and extreme coldness. Secondarily treats abdominal pain, spermatorrhea, and diarrhea.

Ban Xia

Ban Xia mainly treats vomiting due to phlegm-fluids. Secondarily treats pain in the heart, acid reflux, pain in the throat, cough, palpitation, and borborygmus.

Xiao Ban Xia Tang and Wu Ling San have similar indications. Xiao Ban Xia Tang treats vomiting with phlegm fluids while Wu Ling San treats vomiting with inhibited urination.

Wu Wei Zi

Wu Wei Zi mainly treats cough with veiling sensation.

Wu Wei Zi and Ze Xie both treat veiling sensation, but there is difference between the two. Wu Wei Zi treats veiling sensation with cough, whereas Ze Xie treats veiling sensation with dizziness.

Gua Lou Shi

Gua Lou Shi mainly treats focal distention in the chest, and secondarily treats phlegm fluids.

Ge Gen

Ge Gen mainly treats stiffness in the nape and back. Secondarily treats panting and sweating.

Fang Ji

Fang Ji mainly treats water.

Mu Fang Ji Tang treats water with distention and hardness below the heart since its king herb is Ren Shen. Fang Ji Fu Ling Tang treats water abscess with trembling of limbs since Fu Ling is the king herb. Fang Ji Huang Qi Tang treats water abscess with sweating and heaviness in the body due to Huang Qi as a king herb.

Xiang Chi[31]

Xiang Chi mainly treats anguish in the heart. Secondarily treats obstruction and pain in the heart, fullness in the heart and irritability.

Ze Xie

Ze Xie mainly treats inhibited urination and veiling sensation with dizziness. Secondarily treats thirst.

---

[31] It is fermented bean and also referred to as Dan Dou Chi.

Yi Yi Ren

Yi Yi Ren mainly treats edema.

Xie Bai

Xie Bai mainly treats pain in the heart and chest, asthma, cough and phlegm. Secondarily treats distention in the heart and heart pain radiating to the back.

Gan Jiang

Gan Jiang mainly treats obstructed water toxins. Secondarily treats vomiting, cough, diarrhea, extreme coldness, irritability and agitation, pain in the abdomen, chest and low back.

Xing Ren

Xing Ren mainly treats stagnated water in the chest and diaphregm. Therefore it can treat panting and cough. Secondarily treats shortness of breath, obstruction in the chest (Jie Xiong), pain in the heart, and propensity for edema.

Da Zao

Da Zao mainly treats muscle cramps with tightness and a pulling sensation. Secondarily treats cough, palpitation, irritability and agitation, bodyache, pain in the chest and abdomen.

Ju Pi

Ju Pi mainly treats hiccups. Secondarily treats distention in the chest and stagnated phlegm.

Wu Zhu Yu

Wu Zhu Yu mainly treats vomiting with distention of the chest.

Gua Di (瓜蒂)[32]

Gua Di mainly treats toxins in the chest with symptoms of wanting to vomit but not being able to vomit.

Gui Zhi

Gui Zhi mainly treats surging counterflow. Secondarily treats running piglet syndrome, headaches, fever, aversion to wind, sweating and bodyaches.

Hou Po

Hou po mainly treats fullness in the chest and abdomen. Secondarily treats abdominal pain.

Zhi Shi

Zhi Shi mainly treats obstructed toxins. Secondarily treats chest fullness, chest distention, abdominal fullness, and abdominal pain.

Zhi Zi

Zhi Zi mainly treats heart vexation. Secondarily treats jaundice.

Suan Zao Ren

Suan Zao Ren mainly treats irritability and agitation in the chest causing insominia.

---

[32] Cucumeris Melonis Pedicellus. It is melon stalk.

Fu Ling

Fu Ling mainly treats palpitation and trembling of muscles. Secondarily treats inhibited urination, dizziness, irritability and agitation.

Zhu Ling

Zhu Ling mainly treats thirst and inhibited urination.

Long Gu

Long Gu mainly treats pulsation below the navel. Secondarily treats irritability, fright, and spermatorrhea.

Mu Li

Mu Li mainly treats pulsation in the chest and abdominal area. Secondarily treats fright, madness, irritability and agitation.

3. Kokan Igaku(皇漢醫學)

After the Meiji restoration occurred in 1868, the practice of Kampo drastically declined since all Kampo-related systematic education was stopped. The physicians like Dr. Yumoto Kyushin (1876–1942) and Dr. Otsuka Keisetsu (1900-1980) played important role in reviving Kampo medicine.

Especially, <Japanese-Chinese Medicine (Kokan Igaku, 1927)>, written by Dr. Yumoto Kyushin, was the first book on Kampo medicine in which Western medical findings were used to interpret classical Chinese texts[33]. It is a comprehensive text explaining the herbs and formulas of Shang Han Lun along with modern interpretation on

---

[33] Pattern Classification in Kampo Medicine by S. Yakubo, M. Ito, Y. Ueda, H. Okamoto, Y. Kimura, Y. Amano, T. Togo, H. Adachi, T. Mitsuma, and K. Watanabe

each clause, providing comparison of strong and weak points of both Eastern and Western medicine.

Dr. Otsuka Keisetsu, a fourth generation physician, studied with Dr. Yumoto and other several Kampo doctors after inspired by the book, <Kokan Igaku>. He also wrote numerous books to share his knowledge and experience integrating Kampo with the modern medicine. His outstanding interpretation on Shang Han Lun was based mainly on Kang Ping edition of Shang Han Lun, and Kang Ping Shang Han Lun is discussed in Chapter 4.

Chapter 3

Clinical Applications

The common idea shared by Dr. Lee and Dr. Todo is that diseases originate from the state of a person's mind. However, their approaches and methods to improve the diseases are totally opposite in that one focuses on boosting up constitutional weakness and the other on attacking excessive toxins in the body. Dr. Todo didn't believe in the concept of ameliorating a deficiency with herbs.

However, in clinical applications, it is critical to adopt both approaches to prescribe customized herbs for a variety people with numerous conditions. The conventional TCM approach has been mainly based on common physiology of the human body, and while Dr. Todo focused on selecting herbs with respect to specific signs and symptoms, he still based his approach on common physiological perspectives. On the other hand, Dr. Lee's SCM approach is based on individual physiology.

In clinical practice with herbal formulas, it is extremely beneficial to realize which type of person the formula will be applied to rather than only recognizing the disease and symptoms. This is why formulas don't work when we only follow the indications of the formula.

This doesn't mean that Dr. Lee's formulas can treat every condition, which some SCM practitioners might believe. As mentioned in the Chapter 1, it is meaningful that SCM gives four main indicators to approach the human body. However, in clinical practices, there can be a number of variations especially in the modern society where people take tons of medications and supplements, and surgeries and shots are so prevalent.

Here are case studies utilizing the SCM formulas and Shang Han Lun formulas, considering the person's body type and the signs and symptoms of herbs from Shang Han Lun and Jin Gui Yao Lue in addition to the main indications of their formulas.

1. Formula applications for Shao Yin Constitution

Case 1) Ulcerative Colitis and infertility

Female, 36 years old, Persian, 5'4", 122lbs

She is an office manager who has a six year old daughter. For the last couple years, she and her husband tried to conceive a second child, but she could not get pregnant. She has been suffering from ulcerative colitis for more than 10 years, and recently the symptoms has gotten worse causing abdominal distention and pain, rectal bleeding, gas, and borborygmus. On palpation, her epigastrium and lower abdomen areas were tender to the touch.

She is gentle and calm, with a slim body, soft fair skin, cold hands and feet, and well developed hip area. She also experiences chronic fatigue, IBS and indigestion. All of these presentations constitute a classic picture of the Shao Yin Body type.

The SCM formula, Xiang Sha Yang Wei Tang was prescribed. After taking the formula for 2-3 weeks, her pain in the abdomen and the rectal bleeding stopped. However, when her periods started, she had unusually dark heavy bleeding with abdominal cramps. After explaining that these initial hardships could be part of a cleansing process or a sign that her body was not quite ready for pregnancy, The same formula was given for four more weeks.

A few months later, she came in with a ultrasound picture of twins. And in about a year, she brought me a picture of twin boys. She was very happy that these boys were born very healthy, as her first daughter had to have a surgery for a birth defect, a cleft lip.

Case 2) Benign Prostate Hyperplasia (BPH)

Male, 63 years old, Caucasian, 5'10", 171lbs

He had been experiencing frequent urination, with symptoms worsening over the past year and was recently diagnosed with BPH. He stated that he wanted to try something more natural before starting medications.

He is a calm and mellow gentleman who also was experiencing chronic fatigue from a cazy schedule working in the film industry and the frequent urination waking him at night. He tends to get cold easily and has cold hands and feet. He is slim and has a larger hip area, at least for a man. He also complained of low sexual drive and delayed ejaculation. On palpation, no areas of his abdomen were tender to the touch.

The SCM formula, Bu Zhong Yi Qi Tang, was prescribed. After 5 weeks of taking this formula, he was able to sleep through the night, and his energy and sensitivity to cold was improved. The stream of urine was also improved during the day, but the flow of his initial urination in the morning was still slow.

The Shang Han Lun formula, Gui Zhi Jia Fu Zi Tang, was given for 3 more weeks, and his urine stream was all better, and the exam for the BPH turned out to be normal.

Case 3) Ocular Migraine

Female, 29 years old, Caucasian, 5'6", 125lbs

She is a high school teacher and has migraine headaches with aura and visual obstruction every month right before periods. They always affect only her left eye. She also suffers from menstrual cramps and premenstrual syndrome exemplified by mood swings, breast tenderness, bloating, and fatigue. Occasionally she also gets pollen induced allergies with sneezing, white phlegm, itchy eyes, and mild wheezing.

Her skin is soft and resilient, her hands and feet are cold to the touch, and her hip area is well developed. She is very calm and reserved. The SCM formula of Xiang Fu Zi Ba Wu Tang[34] (*Eight Noble Ingredients Decoction with Cyperus*) was prescribed. It is specifically for Shaoyin woman's stress related symptoms including dull headaches, anxiety, and dry throat and tongue.

After taking this formula for 3 weeks, she noticed her overall symptoms were improved around her periods. She continued taking the formula for 8 more weeks, and her ocular migraines were completely gone.

---

[34] Xiang Fu 8, Dang Gui 8, Bai Shao 8, Bai Zhu 4, He Shou Wu 4, Chuan Xiong 4, Chen Pi 4, Zhi Gan Cao 4, Sheng Jiang 4, Da Zao 4

Case 4) Sciatic Neuritis

Female, 15 years old, Caucasian,, 4'11", 99lbs

This adorable 15 year old girl loves ballet and practices at least 3 hours everyday. Too much repetitive motion has caused her back pain radiating down to the left hip, and it was recommended she stop practicing for a few weeks. She was diagnosed with sciatic neuritis. Aleve helped, but her pain came back when she stopped taking it.

She has soft and fair skin with cold hands and feet. She feels cold easily and frequently experiences indigestion with nausea. She stated that she had slightly yellow sputum every morning. All signs and symptoms indicate that she is a Shaoyin with a weak spleen, except that she has a less developed hip area. This could be due to her body not being fully developed, or her not fitting the Shao Yin body type completely.

The Shang Han Lun formula, Xiao Chai Hu Tang, was given to her first for a couple weeks, and nausea, phlegm, and her back and hip pain were gone. She was able to go back to ballet practice again. However, the hip flexor muscle got tight and painful with practice, and Gui Zhi Tang was prescribed. The hip flexors were then loosened and she was able to practice ballet without any discomfort.

Case 5) Adhesive capsulitis

Male, 63 years old, Caucasian, 5'9", 167lbs

He is a golf instructor. He has had shoulder pain on and off, and recently the pain has gotten worse and the ROM of his right shoulder was limited to 30 degrees in abduction. On observation, both of his hands trembled noticeably. The muscles of his shoulders were tight due to golf practice. He is tall, slim, and well proportioned. Ling Gui Gan Zao Tang was prescribed. After taking this formula for a week, he stopped by to leave a message to cancel the next treatment since his shoulder felt all better.

Case 6) Osteoarthritis and degenerative disc disease

Female, 67 years old, Caucasian,, 5'4", 121lbs

She came in for joint pain in both her hands. It was severe debilitating pain that was excruciating at times and put her on disability. She was diagnosed with osteoarthritis and found that her cartilage was worn out. She couldn't do most of her daily activities due to the constant pain and she was scared of attacks of excruciating pain. However, she couldn't take medications due to allergic reactions. The lists of the medicine that she was allergic to include Triamcinolone, Amoxicillin, Azithromycin, Clindamycin Hydrochloride, Diamox, Lisinopril, Mobic, Naproxin, Sulfa, and Tetracyclines Class.

On observation, her metacarpal phalangeal joints had developed moderate deformity on both hands. Her hands and feet are cold to the touch. Her skin is fair and soft. Her body is proportionally well balanced. She suffers from chronic fatigue and has high blood pressure from time to time. She also experiences dizziness and breathing difficulty at high altitude.

The formula of *Jin Gui Yao Lue,* Ling Gui Wei Gan Tang, was prescribed. After taking this formula for a month, her pain subsided and she was able to do chores around house.

A couple month later, she came in for low back pain diagnosed as degenerative disc disease at L4-5 and moderate thoracolumbar scoliosis. The same formula was prescribed to her and the back pain was diminished.

Case 7) Lumbar Radiculopathy

Female, 63 years old, Caucasian,, 5'8", 149lbs

She had worked at a government office for about 30 years and recently retired, earlier than her original plan, to help take care of her grandson. 2 weeks ago, back pain started out of nowhere without any injury or accident, and has gradually gotten worse. It was mainly left back pain radiating down the side of her leg to the front of her left foot. The extreme pain made her body tilt 30 degrees and she limped when she walked and had to use cane. She took hydrocodone but it didn't work. She stated that she had occasional arm pain only in extreme cold in the winter, but never had back pain before. She also felt a cold sensation in the left foot with severe pain and numbness and couldn't sleep at night due to the pain.

The Shang Han Lun formula, Gui Zhi Qu Shao Yao Tang, was prescribed 3 times a day. Her pain gradually diminished each day. After about three weeks, she was able to stand straight, sleep better, and the cold sensation and numbness in her left foot also improved.

Case 8) Joint pain with sciatica

Female, 49 years old, Asian(Filipino), 5'2", 137lbs

This patient has had joint pain for years, and this year it has gotten much worse. Affected areas include shoulders, elbows, wrists, upper back, hips, knees and ankles. The pain is so severe that she cannot lay still during treatment and can't sleep at night. She was so sensitive to needles that she wanted to have only cupping and herbal formulas. She stated that she had had Kidney stones a few years ago.

Her lower body was slightly more developed than the upper, but overall well balanced. Her skin is slightly darker, soft and resilient. She tends to feel cold easily and cold aggrevates her pain. She sweats easily, especially in her hands. She cannot drink milk because it causes stomachache.

The Shang Han Lun formula, Gui Zhi Jia Fu Zi Tang, was prescribed. After taking this formula for a month, her extreme pain was calmed, she was able to sleep at night, and her hands were not as sweaty as before. She continued taking the formula 6 more weeks and didn't have to come back.

Case 9) Tourette Syndrome

Male, 15 years old, Caucasian, 5'4", 105lbs

His mom brought him in because he was suffering from Tourette Syndrome. The main symptom was yelling and screaming at night. His body was thin and his hands and feet were cold to the touch. On abdominal palpation, there was pulsation felt left of the navel. He stated that he had been anxious and occasionally experienced twitching eyes. His urination and bowel movement were normal. The Shang Han Lun formula, Chai Hu Jia Long Gu Mu Li Tang, (without Da Huang) was given to him for a couple of weeks. He came in and stated that he didn't wake up yelling and screaming, but he didn't like the taste of herbal formula and discontinued.

Case 10) Anxiety and Eczema

Male, 22 years old, Caucasian, 5'8", 159lbs

He recently graduated from UC Berkeley and broke up with his girlfriend. He used to want to go to graduate school but put aside his plan due to anxiety and depression, and returned to his parents' house. He came in with his mom since he is very afraid of driving. His mom said he got a driver's license when his exgirlfriend pushed him to take the test but never wanted to drive himself. He also complained of eczema, poor digestion, bloating, yellow tinged and copious phlegm, and low energy. He was taking an antihistamine for asthma and rashes, and an antacid for acid reflux and heartburn.

He is slim and his upper and lower body are evenly developed. He speaks quietly, showing his reserved nature. He said he feels cold easily and prefers warm weather.

The Shang Han Lun formula, Ban Xia Xie Xin Tang, was prescribed for 4 weeks. He didn't have to take his antacid medicine and overall his mood and digestion was improved. He applied for a teaching assistant position at community college and started working with students. He continued taking the same formula for 3 more weeks, and his eczema was diminished and his phlegm reduced.

Case 11) Dysmenorrhea

Female, 16 years old, Caucasian, 5'5", 124lbs

She came in with her mom, complaining of right shoulder pain radiating down to her elbow. Her mom stated that she seemed to get this pain from playing volleyball. She had tried different therapies for a couple months, but the shoulder pain remained the same. Her secondary complaint was debilitating severe menstrual cramps which prevent her from attending school at least a week per cycle. She had been taking Pamprin and birth control pills, but these didn't work. She also suffered from asthma since childhood, which is under control with the use of an inhaler. She said she had very low energy and copious yellow sputum which bothered her.

She has a slim body with soft fair skin and cold hands and feet. She experienced alternating chills and fever during the day, and the menstrual pain was mainly in her lower abdomen, spreading to the hypochondriac and epigastric area.

The Shang Han Lun formula, Xiao Chai Hu Tang, was prescribed for a week before her periods. She came in the next week and stated that her cramps and arm pain were gone and she was able to attend school. Her phlegm amount was significantly reduced. The same formula was given to her for one more week.

Case 12) Headache and Brachial Neuritis

Female, 43 years old, Hispanic, 5'3", 154lbs

She is a housewife busy taking care of her kids, and her nephews and nieces visiting from Mexico. Her chief complaint is neck and shoulder pain and headache. She was diagnosed with brachial neuritis and had taken Prednisone which made it better, but her primary doctor didn't recommend taking it for too long. She stated she also had been having leg spasms and ankle swelling almost every morning for years. She feels cold very easily and cold weather makes her pain worse. The pain level was 7 to 8 in a scale of 1 to 10, but it could go up to 9 or 10 with excruciating head pain when doing outdoor activities with her kids. Range of motion in the right arm was limited to 30 degrees, and the pain was worse with adduction.

She has darker and resilient skin. She stated that she recently gained some weight around her waist.

The Shang Han Lun formula, Gui Zhi Jia Zhu Fu Tang, was prescribed. Both her leg spasms and the swelling in her ankles have gotten better. In a couple months, she recovered full range of motion and the headache and neck pain were gone. She stated that she had more energy and was able to do more of the activities of daily life.

2. Formula Applications for Shao Yang Constitution

Case 1) Rheumatoid Arthritis

Female, 42 years old, Caucasian, 5'6", 123lbs

She was diagnosed with RA and had been taking Humira for about a couple years which helped keep her condition under control. However, recently she got rashes all over her legs, and her doctor recommended she stop the meds because this could be a side effect. Since stopping Humira, her RA symptoms flared up causing shoulder pain and joint swelling, especially in her right wrist and left ankle. She was limping due to this severe ankle and foot swelling. The range of motion in her neck was limited, especially her rotation to the right.

She has red complexion and tends to feel hot all the time. Her upper body is well developed and her muscles gets tight easily. She is usually perky and her voice is slightly hoarse. At night she cannot sleep deeply due to hot flashes. Although all these manifestations indicate she has a heat condition, her shoulder occasionally gets bothered by cold.

The SCM formula, Jing Fang Xie Bai San, was given to her for a couple months. The rashes on her legs and hot flashes were gone and the swelling in her joints was reduced. She was able to walk without limping. The neck and shoulder pain was minimized. And the ROM in her neck fully recovered.

Her pain management doctor put her on a new medicine, Enbreo. It worked well for reducing the inflammation and swelling in her joints, but her neck and shoulder pain started to come back.

The SCM formula, Jing Fang Di Huang Tang, was prescribed. Her neck and shoulder pain was reduced.

Case 2) Tinnitis

Female, 56 years old, Caucasian, 5'3", 162lbs

She has been suffered from ear ringing for years, which was like constant ocean sound, worse in her left ear. She took medicine for ear ringing, and her sypmtoms were relieved, but she had nightmares every night. Her secondary complaints were back pain, knee pain, and anxiety.

Her muscles are tight and firm over all even though she doesn't exercise much. She is slightly overweight, but her waist area is not overly expanded. Her movement is agile and she is in high spirits even with poor sleep. She doesn't complain of any digestive issues.

Dr. Qian Yi's Liu Wei Di Huang Tang was given for a couple weeks, but no improvement in her tinnitus occurred. The SCM formula, Duo Huo Di Huang Tang, was prescribed for a couple weeks. Most of her symptoms, including tinnitus, back pain, and knee pain were significantly reduced. Zuo Gui Wan, since it is in the same lineage of Liu Wei Di Huang Tang, was given to her for a week, but there was not as much improvement. Since then, she has been taking Duo Huo Di Huang Tang on and off whenever she needs to.

Case 3) Back pain / Knee pain

Male, 45 years old, Hispanic, 5'2", 135lbs

He was working for an aircraft company and his job involved lots of physical labors. His chief complaints were back pain, tingling in his face, and fatigue.

He has fair and firm skin with a well developed upper body. The SCM formula, Jing Fang Di Huang Tang, was given to him for three weeks and all the main symptoms were improved significantly.

In a few months he came in again, this time for his knee pain. He also experienced mild sweating at night. He took the SCM formula, Du Huo Di Huang Tang, for a couple weeks, and the symptoms were gone.

Case 4) Adhesive capsulitis

Female, 52 years old, Caucasian, 5'2", 152lbs

This case is of a business woman who runs a women's clothing store in a big shopping center. She had neck and shoulder pain with limited motion in her right shoulder. Other symptoms included headaches, hip pain, hot flashes, night sweats, sinus infection, and ear infection.

She is active, outgoing, and straight forward. She feels hot all the time and complained of not being able to hug her boyfriend due to heat. She is allergic to gluten, which makes her infection worse.

The SCM formula, Liang Ge San Huo Tang, was prescribed for a month. The range of motion in her right shoulder improved, as did the pain, sinus/ear infections, hot flashes and night sweats.

Case 5) Gout

Male, 51 years old, European and Indian, 5'9", 170lbs

He runs his own business and has to pack products for international delivery. He loves bicycling in his free time. Recently his low back pain started to bother him for a few months and prevented him from doing most of his daily activities.

He has dark skin and toned muscles. He tends to be slightly more warm than cold except for cold in his left foot due to childhood polio. He is calm but cheerful and humorous.

He took the SCM formula, Jing Fang Bai Du San, for a couple weeks. His back condition was improved and he was able to go back to work.

A few months later, he came in for gout in his right foot. He has had gout on and off throughout his life, but this time the inflammation was extreme due to Alcohol intake at a family reunion. The same formula was given to him for a week, and he was pleased that it was gone after three days of taking herbs.

Case 6) Chest obstruction with panting

Male, 21 years old, hispanic, 5'8", 252lbs

He came in for difficulty breathing. He had heavy labored breathing with a suffocated feeling in his chest. At first it seemed to be an asthma attack but there was no wheezing. He stated that he felt poisoned with chemicals at work. He couldn't sleep at night and had profuse sweating. He used to work as a server at a restaurant, but he had to quit because he couldn't memorize the menu. He was on medication for seizures. He stated that he occasionally talked with ghosts at night.

He has dark skin and a corpulent body. He speaks incessantly and he feels hot easily. He is cheerful and said he is very impulsive.

The Shang Han Lun formula, Zhi Shi Zhi Zi Chi Tang, was given to him for a couple days. He felt more suffocation in his chest. Another Shang Han Lun formula, Zhi Zi Chi Tang, was prescribed. His breathing improved to normal.

Case 7) Plantar Fasciitis

Female, 52 years old, Caucasian, 5'2", 152lbs

Her chief complaint was foot pain, more on the left side. She was diagnosed with plantar fasciitis. She had had foot pain on and off for more than ten years. She thought it was because she practiced dancing on a hard floor for a long time due to her profession. She also had sinus allergies and hot flashes at night.

She has fair skin and an intense look in her eyes. She also has a well developed upper body and narrow hips. She tends to be warm more than cold.

The SCM formula, Jing Fang Bai Du San, was given to her for five weeks. She was able to step on her feet without pain and didn't limp when walking.

3. Formula applications for Tai Yin Constitution

Case 1) Back Pain and Swollen Knees

Female, 47 years old, Hispanic, 5'2", 165lbs

She came in with severe excruciating back pain that prevented her from walking straight. She has had back pain on and off for years which recently has worsened to the point where she cannot perform any daily activities. She also suffers from migraine and neck pain, and has had surgery for bilateral carpal tunnel syndrome. She has poor sleep due to this debilitating pain.

She tends to be hot more easily than cold. She is corpulent with thick resilient skin. She gets constipated and thirsty easily. Her trapezius muscle gets tight when she is stressed.

The SCM formula, Qing Fei She Gan Tang[35], was prescribed. This formula is a modification of Re Duo Han Shao Tang, adding Da Huang. Her back pain was reduced after taking this formula for a couple months, and she was able to walk straight and do her daily activities.

She came in a year later with a swollen left knee along with neck and shoulder pain. She was limping and sweating profusely. The SCM formula, Ge Gen Tiao Wei Tang[36] was prescribed. All of her main complaints were resolved.

---

[35] Ge Gen 16, Huang Qin 8, Gao Ben 8, Lai Fu Zi 4, Jie Geng 4, Sheng Ma 4, Bai Zhi 4, Da Huang 4
[36] Ge Gen 16, Lai Fu Zi 8, Jie Geng 4, Wu Wei Zi 4, Mai Men Dong 4, Xing Ren 4, Da Huang 4

Case 2) Progressive Leg Pain and Weakness

Male, 38 years old, Caucasian, 6'1", 213lbs

He is an engineer who works for an airplane manufacturing company. One day he woke up with foot pain, mainly in his left foot. The pain was progressively getting worse and his leg and hip were also affected, causing pain and weakness. He came in limping, aided by a cane and his ex wife. He stated that he has high blood pressure, controlled by blood pressure medication.

He has an expanded waist area with dry fair skin. He has a history of childhood asthma. He tends to feel hot easily and occasionally sweats at night.

The SCM formula, Tiao Wei Cheng Qing Tang for Taiyins, was prescribed for a couple months, and he was able to walk normally and go back to work.

A couple years later he came in for the same complaint, and recovered again with the same formula.

Case 3) Plantar Fasciitis

Male, 64 years old, Hispanic, 5'8", 231lbs

He has been playing golf vigorously since retirement. Recently his foot pain started to bother him when playing and he was diagnosed with plantar fasciitis. The pain was excruciating and burning.

He is corpulent with firm and dark skin. He stated that he gets hot easily and occasionally sweats at night. His urination and bowel movement are normal. The SCM formula, *Tiao Wei Cheng Qing Tang* was given. There was no significant improvement. The SCM formula, *Re Duo Han Shao Tang* was prescribed. After about 4 weeks, both his pain and the burning sensation were diminished, and he was able to play golf without any discomfort.

Case 4) Migraine

Female, 34 years old, African American, 5'7", 182lbs

A lead appointment clerk, she has been suffering from migraine and neck and back pain and spasms on and off for 13 years. The pain has been progressively worse this year. Advil helped and reduced pain for a period of time, but she became immune to its effects. All of her blood tests were normal except for blood sugar, for which she has taken Metformin. She also had PCOS.

She tends to feel hot easily and experiences chronic constipation. She also tends to gain weight easily and her Trapezius muscle is very tight.

The Shang Han Lun formula, Ge Gen Huang Lian Huang Qin Tang, was prescribed. Overall her pain level and tightness were reduced, and the activities of her daily life were improved.

Case 5) Cervical spondylosis and displaced cervical discs

Female, 48 years old, Caucasian, 5'7", 188lbs

She is a business owner running an entertainment company. Her chief complaint was neck pain radiating down to her left shoulder, arm and hand. She stated that she had bulging discs, C6 and C7, and that she had numbness and weakness in her left hand causing her to drop things easily. Her neck pain often radiates up, causing headaches. She takes Advil every night before sleep to prevent severe headaches. She stated that she has had gallstones and kidney stones. Her kidney stone analysis showed that it was due to green vegetables, so she has avoided eating green vegetables since then. Her secondary complaint was edema in her ankles, which was not improved with diuretic medicines. She tends to feel cold easily and tired due to hypothyroid. She also suffered from constipation. On palpation her Trapezius was very tight and tender to the touch.

The SCM formua, Han Duo Re Shao Tang, was employed for three weeks, and the swelling in her ankeles was reduced and her energy level was improved. She stated that she had more sensation in her left hand and was able to grab things better without dropping.

However, her headache was not improved. The SCM formula, Ge Gen Jie Ji Tang for Taiyins, was given for a couple weeks. Her headache started to improve and she was able to reduce the dosage of Advil.

Case 6) Bell's Palsy

Female, 51 years old, Caucasian, 5'6", 164lbs

Her boyfriend brought her in for her facial paralysis, which had been bothering her for a month. She cannot close her eyes, with worse symptoms on her left side. Her eyes get watery, especially when it is windy outside.

She tends to feel cold easily. She has an expanded waist area and her skin is fair and slightly loose.

The SCM formula, Tai Yin Tiao Wei Tang, was prescribed for about 7 weeks. She was then able to close her eyes and most of the sensation on her face returned. She was able to leave for a cruise to Europe with her boyfriend.

Case 7) Lumbar Stenosis

Male, 61 years old, Caucasian, 5'5", 187lbs

He is a speed skating coach and real estate agent who won a national championship gold medal in his 20s. He came in for severe back pain diagnosed as spinal stenosis. He could not turn to the side and it was hard for him to walk. He stated that his back pain started after taking medicine for an enlarged prostate (finasteride). He was recommended to have back surgery and had to stop coaching speed skating.

He recently gained more weight especially around his waist due to lack of exercise. He stated that he feels cold very easily. Occasionally he experiences bloating and acid reflux when he doesn't eat foods that agree with him. He also complained of numbness in his feet.

The Shang Han Lun formula, Ma Huang Jia Zhu Fu Tang, was given to him for about four months. He gained full range of motion and was free from back pain. He went back to coaching speed skating and hosted the California State Championship. He took the same formula for 3 more months and the numbness in his feet also disappeared.

Case 8) Anovulation

Female, 32 years old, Caucasian, 5'4", 210lbs

She initially came in for headaches, which were improved with acupuncture treatments. After a few sessions, she stated that she had her regular period but there was no ovulation, causing infertility. She was taking an iron supplement due to low levels of iron. She had her Gall bladder removed due to gall stones last year, and had her tonsils removed when she was 8. She was overweight and had constipation. She tends to feel hot easily. Her skin is fair and soft.

The Shang Han Lun formula, Tao Ren Cheng Qi Tang, was employed for her anovulation. After taking for about a month, she checked her ovulation and it was positive. In her next cycle, she got pregnant. Her other symptoms including headaches and constipation were improved as well.

Case 9) Headaches

Female, 50 years old, Hispanic, 5'4", 178lbs

She is a housewife who has headaches for about 15 years due to an arteriovenous malformation. Her face had an almost permanent frown due to severe headaches in her temporal and occipital area. Her medical history includes but is not limited to visual field defects, a total hysterectomy, acid reflux, tinea pedis, radiation necrosis of central nervous system, bilateral incipient cataract, atropic vaginitis, hyperlipidemia, anxiety, and panic attacks.

She stated that she feels warmer at night and has Charley horse in her calf every morning. Her Trapezius is very tight and tender to the touch. She is obese and her abdominal muscles lack resilience.

The Shang Han Lun formula, Ge Ge Tang, was given to her for 3 weeks. Her headache and muscle tension and spasms were reduced. The same formula was administered for two more weeks, and the deep frown in her face dissipated.

Case 10) Complex Regional Pain Syndrome

Female, 35 years old, Caucasian, 5'5", 131lbs

She came in with left dorsal foot pain that has been consistent for the last three years since foot surgery. She stated that she had been walking better after surgery, but the skin on the top of left foot got extremely sensitive even with very light touch that she couldn't even shower in a normal way since then. Her doctor gave her a referral for acupuncture concerning the healing process is too slow.

On interrogation, her overall condition is good and there are no other symptoms besides this left foot pain. Acupucture treatment for her had to be minimal due to her claustrophobia and hypersensitivity of her foot.

She didn't have any preference between hot and cold temperature. Her skin is slightly firmer side and she didn't have any allergy to any food. She stated that no medication helped reducing her pain.

The SCM formula, *Han Duo Re Shao Tang* was prescribed for about three weeks. She gladly said that she was able to take a normal shower

4. Formula Applications for Tai Yang Constitution

Dr. Lee, in his book *Dongui Suse Bowon*(東醫┌世保元), stated that there are 50% of people are Taiyins, 30% Shaoyangs, 20% Shaoyins, while Taiyangs are very rare. Recent research in Korea has shown that among Koreans 39.2% are Taiyins, 33.7% Shaoyangs, 27.1% Shaoyins, and almost none are Taiyangs. This research was conducted from 2007 to 2014 based on more than four thousand patients whose body types were identified with SCM prescription, and was released in 'BMC Complementary and Alternative Medicine' in March 2015.

In the US, Taiyangs are still rare, and certain ingredients of the Taiyang formula are unavailable, making it hard to prepare these formulas. So, treatments for Taiyangs are mainly composed of acupuncture and nutritional recommendations. Constitutional Acupuncture will be discussed in a separate book. The recommended foods and herbs are green leafy vegetables, buckwheat, clams, crab, squid, octopus, green grape, cherry, persimmon, pine tree leaf, pine pollen, Mu Gua (quince), and Song Jie (pine tree branch). Meat and spicy fatty greasy foods need to be avoided.

Chapter 4

Kang Ping Shang Han Lun

The *Shang Han Lun,* known in English as the *Treatise on Cold Damage Disorders*, is a Chinese medical treatise that was compiled by Dr. Zhang Zhongjing sometime before the year 220 at the end of the Han dynasty. However, the original was almost lost due to conflict, and was later transcribed by Wang Shu He who probably added to original but did not alter the main body text. The Shang Han Lun we know has thus come down to us from Wang Shu He's copy.

There are about a dozen different surviving editions. Among them there are four relatively well known editions, which are the Song dynasty edition, Cheng Wu-chi's Annotated Shang Han Lun, the Jin Gui Yu Han ching, and the Kang Ping edition.

Regarding the Kang Ping edition, Kang Ping is the name of the period from 1058-1068 in the Heian era in Japan. It is the definitive edition and indispensable for study because it retains the ancient style and preserves the classic style of the Jin dynasty. It was accidently found in a Tokyo bookstore by Dr. Otsuka Keisetsu in 1936. After carefully studying the book, he realized that the preface, dated 1060 and written by Tamba Masatata, a famous physician, indicated that it was a Kang Ping edition. It thus preceded the Song dynasty. At that time, therefore, the Kang Ping edition must have been available in Japan, five years before the Song edition was written.

In the study of Shang Han Lun, the editions from the Song dynasty have been the most commonly read among students in Traditional Oriental Medical education. However, since Dr. Todo's study was introduced, Korean practitioners have started to pay attention to the Kang Ping edition, forming a new study trend of Shang Han Lun.

Since it is closest to the original, the Kang Ping edition is more concise, whereas most other editions have additional interpretations such as pulse identification and pulses in normal persons. It is also easier to understand since it is written in three different styles, namely, fifteen-word lines, fourteen-word lines, and thirteen word lines. And it is found that the fifteen-word lines deliver the most important messages of the *Shang Han Lun*.

Here is Kang Ping Shang Han Lun, mainly with fifteen-word lines translated. It is also translated in an effort of delivering the meaning more accurately by distinguishing big letters from small letters as in the original text.

辨太陽病 (Tai Yang Disorders I)

1-1. 太陽之爲病 脈浮 頭項强痛而惡寒. (1)

In Tai Yang Disorder, the pulse is floating, the head and nape are stiff and painful, and there is aversion to cold.

1-2. 太陽病 發熱 汗出 惡風 脈緩者 名爲中風. (2)

In Tai Yang Disorder, when there is fever and sweating, aversion to wind, and the pulse is moderate, it is called 'Zhong Feng (wind attack).'

1-3. 太陽病 或已發熱 或未發熱 必惡寒 體痛 嘔逆 脈陰陽俱緊者 名曰傷寒. (3)

Tai Yang disorder, whether there is fever or no fever, as long as there is an aversion to cold with body pain, nausea, and both the yin and yang pulses are tight, is called 'Shang Han (cold damage).'

1-4. 太陽病 發熱而渴 不惡寒者 爲溫病 若發汗已 身灼熱者 名風溫風溫爲病,脉陰陽俱浮,自汗出,身重,多眠睡,鼻息必鼾,語言難出

In Tai Yang Disorder, if there is fever and thirst without aversion to cold, this is called 'Wen Bing (warm disorder)'. If there is body scorching heat after sweating, this is called wind-warmth. In wind warmth disorder, there are yin and yang pulses, both floating, spontaneous sweating, generalized heaviness, sleepiness, snoring, and difficulty in speech.

1-5. 太陽中風 脈陽浮而陰弱 ^{陽浮者 熱自發 陰弱者 汗自出} 嗇嗇惡寒 淅淅惡風 翕翕發熱 鼻鳴乾嘔者 桂枝湯主之. (12)

In Tai Yang Zhong Feng, the pulse is floating in the superficial level (yang) and weak in the deep level (yin). The floating pulse reflects spontaneous heat effusion, and the weak pulse reflects spontaneous sweating. If there is aversion to cold, aversion to wind, persistent fever, nasal congestion with noisy breathing, or dry retching, Gui Zhi Tang should be used.

1-6. 太陽病 頭痛 發熱 汗出 惡風者 桂枝湯主之. (13)

Gui Zhi Tang primarily treats Tai Yang disorder with headache, fever, sweating, and aversion to cold.

1-7. 太陽病 項背強几几 反汗出惡風者 桂枝加葛根湯主之. (14)

In Tai Yang disorder, when the nape and the back are stiff and tight with sweating, and there is an aversion to wind, Gui Zhi Jia Ge Gen Tang shoud be prescribed.

1-8. 太陽病 下之後 其氣上衝者 可與桂枝湯 (15)

喘家作 桂枝湯加厚朴杏子佳. (18) 又服桂枝湯吐者 其後必吐膿血也. (19)

Gui Zhi Tang also can be used for Tai Yang disorder that has been treated with purging method causing upward counterflow to the chest. For cases of respiratory disorders Gui Zhi Tang can be modified by adding Hou Po and Xing Zi. If a person vomits after taking Gui Zhi Tang, later he or she will vomit pus and blood.

1-9. 太陽病 發汗 遂漏不止 其人惡風 小便難 四肢微急 難以屈伸者 桂枝加附子湯主之. (20)

In Tai Yang disorder, after sweating is induced, when there is incessant perspiration, aversion to wind, urinary difficulty, mild muscle spasms of limbs that leads difficulty in flexion and extension, Gui Zhi Jia Fu Zi Tang governs.

1-10. 太陽病 下之後 脈促胸滿者 桂枝去芍藥湯主之. (21) 若微寒者 桂枝去芍藥加附子湯主之. (22)

After Tai Yang disorder is treated with the purging method, if there is abrupt pulse and fullness in the chest, Gui Zhi Qu Shao Yao Tang should be used. If there is minute pulse and aversion to cold, Gui Zhi Qu Shao Yao Jia Fu Zi Tang governs.

1-11. 太陽病 得之八九日 如瘧狀 發熱惡寒 熱多寒少 其人不嘔 清便欲自可 一日二三
度發. 以其不能得少汗出 身必癢 宜桂枝麻黃各半湯. (23)

In Tai Yang disorder which has been present for eight to nine days, when there are malaria like symptoms of fever and chills (fever more pronounced than chills), no nausea, normal bowel movement, alternating chills and fever two to three times per day, and pruritis without perspiration, Gui Zhi Ma Huang Ge Ban Tang can be applied.

1-12. 太陽病初服桂枝湯 反煩不解者 先刺風池 風府 却與桂枝湯則愈. (24) 服桂枝湯 大汗
出 脈洪大者 與桂枝湯 如前法 若形如瘧 一日再發者 汗出必解 宜桂枝二麻黃一
湯. (25)

If in Tai Yang disorder the symptoms are not resolved even after the first administration of Gui Zhi Tang, acupuncture points GB20 and Du20 need to be needled. Then Gui Zhi Tang can be given again to make it effective. If there is profuse sweating and flooding pulse after taking Gui Zhi Tang, the same formula can be administered again as in previous methods. If there are malaria like symptoms, relapsing twice per day, it is necessary to induce sweating to recover. Gui Zhi Er Ma Huang Yi Tang can be used.

1-13. 服桂枝湯 大汗出後 大煩渴不解 脈洪大者 白虎加人參湯主之. (26)

If there is profuse sweating after taking Gui Zhi Tang that leads to persistent severe thirst and irritability with flooding and big pulse, Bai Hu Jia Ren Shen Tang should be used.

1-14. 太陽病 發熱惡寒 熱多寒少 脈微弱者此無陽也 不可大發汗 宜桂枝二越婢一湯. (27)
服桂枝湯 或下之 仍頭項強痛 翕翕發熱 無汗 心下滿微痛 小便不利者 桂枝去桂
加茯苓白朮湯主之. (28)

When in Tai Yang disorder there are fever and chills (more fever than chills) and minute and weak pulse, it is not recommended to strongly induce sweating due to lack of Yang. Then Gui Zhi Er Yue Bi Yi Tang can be used. If there are headaches, stiffness in the neck, persistent fever without sweating, epigastric fullness with mild pain, and urinary difficulty after either administration of Gui Zhi Tang or purging method, Gui Zhi Qu Gui Jia Fu Ling Bai Zhu Tang governs.

1-15. 傷寒 脈浮 自汗出 小便數 心煩 微惡寒 脚攣急 反與桂枝湯 _{欲攻其表 此誤也} 得之便厥 咽中乾躁 吐逆者 作甘草乾薑湯與之 _{以復其陽}. 若厥愈 足溫者 更作芍藥甘草湯與之. 若胃氣不和 譫語者 小與調胃承氣湯. 若重發汗 復加燒針得之者 回逆湯主之.(29)

When in Shang Han condition there is floating pulse, spontaneous sweating, frequent urination, irritability, mild chills, spasm in the legs, Gui Zhi Tang is not recommended as it might cause frigid limbs, dryness in the throat, irritability, and vomiting. Gan Cao Gan Jiang Tang can be used for the case. If frigid limbs are recovered and feet get warm due to recovered Yang, Shao Yao Gan Cao Tang can be prescribed. If there are stomach disorders and delirious speech, a mild dosage of Tiao Wei Cheng Qi Tang can be administered. If sweating has been induced repeatedly and fire needle is added, Si Ni Tang governs.

辨太陽病 (Tai Yang Disorders II)

2-1. 太陽病 項背強几几 無汗 惡風 葛根湯主之. (31)

Ge Gen Tang governs Tai Yang disorder with stiff nape and back, absence of sweating, and aversion to cold.

2-2. 太陽與陽明合病者 必自下利 葛根湯主之. (32)

In Tai Yang and Yang Ming combination disorder, there will be diarrhea, and Ge Gen Tang governs.

2-3. 太陽與陽明合病 不下利 但嘔者 葛根加半夏湯主之. (33)

In Tai Yang and Yang Ming combination disorder, when there is no diarrhea and only nausea present, Ge Gen Jia Ban Xia Tang governs.

2-4. 太陽病 桂枝證 醫反下之 利遂不止_{脈促者 表未解也} 喘而汗出者 葛根黃連黃芩湯主之. (34)

When in Tai Yang disorder the purging method has been mistakenly used for Gui Zhi Tang pattern, it can lead to diarrhea, abrupt pulse due to unresolved exterior, panting and sweating. Ge Gen Huang Lian Huang Qin Tang governs.

2-5. 太陽病 頭痛發熱 身疼腰痛 骨節疼痛 惡風 無汗而喘者 麻黃湯主之. (35)

When in Tai Yang disorder there are headaches, fever, generalized pain, lumbar pain, joint pain, aversion to cold, absence of sweating, and panting, Ma Huang Tang governs.

○ 太陽與陽明合病 喘而胸滿者 不可下 宜麻黃湯. (36)

In Tai Yang and Yang Ming combination disorder, the purging method cannot be used when there is panting and fullness in the chest. Ma Huang Tang is appropriate.

○ 太陽病 十日以去 脈浮細而嗜臥者 外已解也 設胸滿脅痛者 與小柴胡湯 脈但浮者 與麻黃湯. (37)

After ten days of Tai Yang disorder where there is floating and thready pulse and somnolence, it means the exterior has already resolved. If there is fullness in the chest and hypochondriac pain, give Xiao Chai Hu Tang. If there is only floating pulse, give Ma Huang Tang.

2-6. 太陽中風 脈浮緊 發熱惡寒 身疼痛 不汗出而煩躁者 大青龍湯主之 若脈微弱 汗出 惡風者 不可服之 服之則厥逆 此爲逆也 筋惕肉瞤. (38)

When in the Zhong Feng condition of Tai Yang disorder there is floating tight pulse, fever, chills, generalized aches and pain, absence of sweating, irritability, Da Qing Long Tang governs. If the pulse is minute and weak and there is sweating and aversion to cold, this formula is contraindicated as it may cause frigid limbs and twitching of sinews and muscles.

2-7. 傷寒脈浮緩 身不疼 但重 乍有輕時 無少陽證者 大青龍湯主之. (39)

Da Qing Long Tang should be used for Shang Han condition with floating moderate pulse, no generalized pain, and only heaviness with occasional lightness.

2-8. 傷寒表不解 心下有水氣 乾嘔發熱而咳 或渴 或利 或噎 小便不利 少腹滿 或喘者 小青龍湯主之. (40)

In Shang Han condition when the exterior has not resolved and there is water accumulation in the epigastric area, dry retching, fever, and cough, possibly thirst, or diarrhea, or dysphagia, urinary difficulty, fullness in the lower abdomen, or panting, Xiao Qing Long Tang governs.

2-9. 傷寒 心下有水氣 咳而微喘 發熱不渴 _{服湯已渴者 此寒去欲解也} 小青龍湯主之. (41)

When in Shang Han condition, there is water accumulation in the epigastric area, cough, mild panting, fever, no thirst, Xiao Qing Long Tang governs. Thirst after taking this formula means the cold pathogen has been removed and is about to resolve.

2-10. 太陽病 外證未解 脈浮弱者 當以汗解 宜桂枝湯. (42)

In Tai Yang disorder when the exterior pattern has not resolved and there is floating weak pulse, it is necessary to induce sweating by using Gui Zhi Tang.

2-11. 太陽病 下之微喘者 表未解故也 桂枝加厚朴杏子湯主之. (43)

In Tai Yang disorder, mild panting after inappropriate purgation means the exterior has not resolved. Gui Zhi Jia Hou Pou Xing Zi Tang governs.

2-12. 太陽病 外證未解 不可下 _{下之爲逆} 欲解外者 宜桂枝湯. (44)

In Tai Yang disorder when the exterior pattern has not resolved, the purging method cannot be used as it is an adverse treatment. To release the exterior, Gui Zhi Tang is appropriate.

◯ 太陽病 先發汗不解 而復下之 脈浮者不愈 浮爲在外 而反下之 故令不愈 今脈浮 故在外 當須解外則愈 宜桂枝湯. (45)

In Tai Yang disorder, when the exterior has not resolved after inducing perspiration and the purging method is applied, floating pulse means the person has not recovered because floating pulse indicates the pathogen still exists on the exterior.

So, if the purging method is used adversely, the disease cannot be resolved. Gui Zhi Tang is appropriate to release exterior and hasten recovery.

2-13. 太陽病 脈浮緊 無汗 發熱 身疼痛 八九日不解 表證仍在 _{此當發其汗 服藥已 微除也} 其人發 煩 目瞑 劇者必衄 _{乃愈} 所以然者 陽氣重故也 麻黃湯主之. (46)

When Tai Yang disorder with floating and tight pulse, absence of sweating, fever, and generalized pain has not resolved in eight or nine days, it indicates that the exterior pattern is still present. This can be improved with the formula to induce sweating. If the person also suffers from irritability, dizziness, and in severe cases epistaxis (symptoms are resolved thereafter), it is due to Yang Qi being heavy. Ma Huang Tang governs.

○ 脈浮者 病在表 可發汗 宜麻黃湯. (51)

Floating pulse indicates that the disease is in the exterior. Sweating can be promoted, and Ma Huang Tang is appropriate.

○ 脈浮而數者 可發汗 宜麻黃湯. (52)

Floating rapid pulse indicates that sweating can be induced. Ma Huang Tang is appropriate.

病常自汗出者 此爲榮氣和 榮氣和者 外不諧 以衛氣不共榮氣諧和故爾 以榮行脈中 衛 行脈外 復發其汗 榮衛和則愈 宜桂枝湯. (53)

When disease is characterized by spontaneous sweating, it means nutritive qi is in harmony but the exterior is not. It also means that defensive qi is not in harmony with nutritive qi. Since nutritive qi runs in the vessels and defensive qi runs outside the vessels, further inducing perspiration can harmonize them and lead to recovery. Gui Zhi Tang is appropriate.

○ 病人 藏無他病 時發熱 自汗出而不愈者 此衛氣不和也 先其時發汗則愈 宜桂枝湯. (54)

When a patient has no other disease in the organs but has fever, spontaneous sweating, and is not recovered, it is due to disharmony in defensive qi. Promote sweating first and recovery will be obtained. Gui Zhi Tang is appropriate.

2-14. 傷寒脈浮緊 不發汗 因致衄者 麻黃湯主之. (55)

When in Shang Han condition with floating tight pulse sweating is not promoted, it can lead to nosebleeds. Ma Huang Tang governs.

◯ 傷寒不大便 六七日 頭痛有熱者 與承氣湯 其小便清者 知不在裏 仍在表也 當須發汗 若頭痛者 必衄 宜桂枝湯. (56)

Shang Han condition with inability to defecate for six to seven days, headache, and fever can be treated with Cheng Qi Tang. If the urine is clear, it means that the disease is not in the interior but is still in the exterior and it is necessary to promote sweating. If there are headaches, there will be nosebleeds. Gui Zhi Tang is appropriate.

傷寒發汗已解 半日許 復煩 脈浮數者 可更發汗 宜桂枝湯. (57)

In Shang Han condition treated by the promotion of sweating where exterior has been resolved, if a half day passes and there again occurs irritability and floating and rapid pulse, it is recommended to induce sweating again. Gui Zhi Tang is appropriate.

發汗後 身疼痛 脈沈遲者 桂枝加芍藥生薑各一兩人參三兩新加湯主之. (62)

After sweating is promoted, when there is generalized pain and deep and slow pulse, Gui Zhi Jia Shao Yao Sheng Jiang Ge Yi Liang Ren Shen San Liang Xin Jia Tang governs.

發汗後 喘家不可更行桂枝湯 汗出而喘 無大熱者 可與麻黃杏仁甘草石膏湯. (63)

After sweating is promoted, when there is panting and wheezing, Gui Zhi Tang cannot be used again. For those who have sweating and panting with mild fever, Ma Huang Xing Ren Gan Cao Shi Gao Tang can be used.

◯ 發汗過多 其人叉手自冒心 心下悸 欲得按者 桂枝甘草湯主之. (64)

After excessive promotion of sweating, when the person covers the heart with his/her hands and there are palpitations in the epigastric area, Gui Zhi Gan Cao Tang governs.

◯ 發汗後 其人臍下悸者 欲作奔豚 茯苓桂枝甘草大棗湯主之. (65)

After the promotion of sweating, when the person has palpitations below the navel about to become running piglet, Fu Ling Gui Zhi Gan Cao Da Zao Tang governs.

發汗後 腹脹滿者 厚朴生薑半夏甘草人參湯主之. (66)

After sweating is promoted, when there is abdominal bloating and distention, Hou Po Sheng Jiang Ban Xia Gan Cao Ren Shen Tang governs.

2-15. 傷寒 若吐若下後 心下逆滿 氣上衝胸 起則頭眩 脈沈緊 發汗則動經 身爲振振搖者 茯苓桂枝白朮甘草湯主之. (67)

After Shang Han condition is treated adversely with vomiting and purging methods, epigastric counterflow fullness, qi surging upward to chest, dizziness upon standing, and deep and tight pulse all can occur. If sweating is promoted, the meridians will be disturbed causing trembling of the body. Fu Ling Gui Zhi Bai Zhu Gan Cao Tang governs.

發汗 病不解 反惡寒者 虛故也 芍藥甘草附子湯主之. (68)

When after sweating is promoted and the disease is still not resolved but there is aversion to cold, Shao Yao Gan Cao Fu Zi Tang governs.

發汗若下之 病仍不解 煩躁者 茯苓回逆湯主之. (69)

After sweating is promoted, if the purging method is used and the disease is still not resolved, and there is irritability, Fu Ling Si Ni Tang governs.

發汗後 惡寒者 虛故也 不惡寒 但熱者 實也 當和胃氣 與調胃承氣湯. (70)

After sweating is promoted, if there is aversion to cold, it is due to deficiency. If there is no aversion to cold but is only fever, it is excess. For the excess, it is necessary to harmonize stomach qi by giving Tiao Wei Cheng Qi Tang.

2-16. 太陽病 發汗後 大汗出 胃中乾 躁煩不得眠 欲將飲水者 少少與飲之 令胃氣和則愈 若脈浮 小便不利 微熱消渴者 五苓散主之. (71)

In Tai Yang disorder, after sweating is promoted, when there is profuse sweating, dryness in the stomach, insomnia with irritability, and desire to drink water, a small sip of water given little by little harmonizes the stomach qi and leads to recovery. If there is floating pulse, urinary difficulty, mild fever, and thirst, Wu Ling San governs.

2-17. 發汗已 脈浮數 煩渴者 五苓散主之. (72)

After the promotion of sweating, when there is floating and rapid pulse, and irritability and thirst, Wu Ling San governs.

2-18. 傷寒 汗出而渴者 五苓散主之 不渴者 茯苓甘草湯主之. (73)

Wu Ling San governs Shang Han condition with sweating and thirst. When there is no thirst, Fu Ling Gan Cao Tang governs.

2-19. 中風發熱 六七日不解而煩 ^{有表裏證} 渴欲飲水 水入口吐者 ^{名曰水逆} 五苓散主之. (74)

Wu Ling San governs Zhong Feng condition in which there is an unresolved fever after six to seven days, irritability, thirst with a desire to drink water, and vomiting after drinking water.

2-20. 發汗後 水藥不得入口^{爲逆} 若更發汗 必吐下不止 發汗吐下後 虛煩不得眠 若劇者 必反復顛倒 心中懊憹 梔子豉湯主之 若少氣者 梔子甘草豉湯主之 若嘔者 梔子生薑豉湯主之. (76)

After inducing sweating, when a person cannot drink water or an herbal decoction, it is due to counterflow. If sweating is induced again, there should be incessant vomiting and diarrhea. After sweating, vomiting, and purging methods are applied, irritability and insomnia will occur. If the condition is severe, repeated tossing and turning and anguish in the heart are expected. Zhi Zi Chi Tang governs. If there is deficiency of Qi, Zhi Zi Gan Cao Chi Tang governs. If there is nausea, Zhi Zi Sheng Jiang Chi Tang governs.

2-21. 發汗 若下之 而煩熱 胸中窒者 梔子豉湯主之. (77)

Zhi Zi Chi Tang governs heat irritability and obstruction in the chest after inducing sweating followed by purgation.

2-22. 傷寒五六日 大下之後 身熱不去 心中結痛者 未欲解也 梔子豉湯主之. (78)

In Shang Han condition that has been present for five to six days, when there remains a lingering fever and pain and obstruction in the heart after strong purgation, Zhi Zi Chi Tang governs.

2-23. 傷寒下後 心煩 腹滿 臥起不安者 梔子厚朴湯主之. (79)

Zhi Zi Hou Po Tang is indicated for irritability, abdominal fullness, and restlessness after purgation for the Shang Han condition.

2-24. 傷寒 醫以丸藥大下之 身熱不去 微煩者 梔子乾薑湯主之. (80)

In Shang Han condition, when the strong-purging method is applied with herbal pills but the generalized fever has not subsided and there is still slight irritability, Zhi Zi Gan Jiang Tang governs.

大下之後 復發汗亡津 小便不利者 勿治之 得小便利 必自愈. (59)

When sweating is induced again after strong purgation, it can cause urinary difficulty, which is due to the collapse of body fluids. Even without any treatment, as long as urination become normal, the person will naturally recover.

下之後 復發汗 必振寒 脈微細 所以然者 以內外俱虛故也. (60)

When sweating is induced again after purgation, there will be trembling and aversion to cold with minute and thready pulse due to both an interior and exterior deficiency.

下之後 發汗 晝日煩躁 不得眠 夜而安靜 不嘔 不渴 無表證 脈沈微 身無大熱者 乾薑附子湯主之. (61)

When sweating is induced again after purgation, there is irritability during the day but not at night, no nausea, no thirst, no exterior symptoms, no generalized high fever, and a deep and minute pulse, Gan Jiang Fu Zi Tang governs.

2-25. 太陽病 發汗 汗出不解 其人仍發熱 心下悸 頭眩 身ⲣ動 振振欲擗地者 玄武湯主之. (82)

When Tai Yang disorder is still not resolved even after perspiration, and a person continues to have fever, palpitation, dizziness, body twitching, trembling, and a tendency to collapse, Zhen Wu Tang governs.

2-26. 傷寒 醫下之 續得下利 清穀不止 身疼痛者 急當救裏 後身疼痛 清便自調者 急當可救表 救裏宜回逆湯 救表宜桂枝湯. (91)

When after the purging method is applied in Shang Han condition, and there is incessant diarrhea with undigested food and generalized pain, it is necessary to treat the interior first before treating the generalized pain. Once the bowel movement is regulated, the exterior can be treated. The interior can be addressed with Si Ni Tang while the exterior with Gui Zhi Tang.

2-27. 太陽病 未解 脈陰陽俱停 下之必先振慄 汗出而解 _{但陽脈微者 汗出而解 但陰脈微者 下之而解} 若欲下之 宜調胃承氣湯. (94)

When Tai Yang disorder has not been resolved and both yin and yang pulses are resting, the purging method will lead to shivering and quivering first, with perspiration then signaling its resolution. If only the yang pulse is minute, perspiration will indicate a resolution. If only the yin pulse is minute, purgation will resolve. If one desires to purge, Tiao Wei Cheng Qi Tang is appropriate.

◯ 太陽病 發熱汗出者 此爲榮弱衛強 故使汗出 欲救邪風者 宜桂枝湯. (95)

Tai Yang disorder with fever and sweating means weakness in Ying and excess in Wei. Therefore Gui Zhi Tang is appropriate to induce sweating and release the evil wind.

2-28. 傷寒五六日 ^{中風} 往來寒熱 胸脇苦滿 ⲅⲅ不欲飲食 心煩 喜嘔 或脇中煩而不嘔 或渴 或腹中痛 或胸下痞硬 或心下悸 小便不利 或不渴 身有微熱 或咳者 小柴胡湯主之. (96)

In Shang Han condition that has been present for five to six days, when Zhong Feng symptoms change to alternating chills and fever, fullness and distention of the chest and hypochondrium, speechlessness and anorexia, irritability and nausea, Xiao Chai

Hu Tang governs. Or if there is irritability with no nausea or thirst, abdominal pain or distention and hardness under the chest, or palpitation and urinary difficulty, or no thirst and mild generalized fever or cough, Xiao Chai Hu Tang also governs.

2-29. 傷寒四五日 身熱 惡風 頸項强 脇下滿 手足溫而渴者 小柴胡湯主之. (99)

In Shang Han condition that has lasted for four to five days, when there is generalized fever, aversion to wind, stiffness in the neck, fullness in the hypochondrium, warm extremities, and thirst, Xiao Chai Hu Tang governs.

2-30. 傷寒 陽脈濇 陰脈弦 法當腹中急痛 □□先與小建中湯 不差者 小柴胡湯主之. (100)

Shang Han condition with choppy pulse in the yang level and wiry pulse in the yin level will have acute abdominal pain that needs to be treated with Xiao Jian Zhong Tang first. If not resolved completely, Xiao Chai Hu Tang should then be used.

2-31. 傷寒二三日 心中悸而煩者 小建中湯主之. (102)

On the second or third day of the Shang Han condition, when there are palpitations and irritability, Xiao Jian Zhong Tang governs.

2-32. 太陽病 過經十餘日 反二三下之 後四 五日 柴胡證仍在者 先與小柴胡湯 嘔不止 心下急 鬱鬱微煩者 爲未解也 與大柴胡湯下之 則愈. (103)

In Tai Yang disorder that had lasted for over ten days, when four to five days have passed since the purging method was applied two to three times in adverse, the Chai Hu Tang pattern may exist. Xiao Chai Hu Tang needs to be applied first. When a person still suffers from incessant nausea, obstruction below the heart, and depression with mild irritability due to unresolved pathogens, Da Chai Hu Tang is applied to purge and will result in recovery.

2-33. 傷寒 十三日不解 胸脇滿而嘔 日晡所發潮熱 已而微利 此本柴胡 下之而不得利 今反利者 知醫以丸藥下之 此非其治也 潮熱者 實也 先宜服小柴胡湯以解外 後以柴胡加芒硝湯主之. (104)

In Shang Han condition that still has not resolved after thirteen days, if there is fullness in the chest and hypochondrium, nausea, tidal fever at sunset, and mild diarrhea, Xiao Chai Hu Tang is appropriate to take initially to release the exterior.

Afterwards Chai Hu Jia Mang Xiao Tang governs. (This is originally the Chai Hu Tang pattern except for the tidal fever, which is part of the excess pattern. Purging method should not cause diarrhea, but if in this case there is diarrhea, it means the purging pill was inappropriately used.)

2-34. 太陽病不解 熱結膀胱 其人如狂 血自下 ^{血自下者 愈} 其外不解者 尚未可攻 當先解其 外 外解已 但小腹急結者 乃可攻之 宜桃核承氣湯. (106)

A person with unresolved Tai Yang disorder and heat obstruction in the bladder will look as if manic. If the obstructed blood descends by itself, there will be recovery. If the exterior has not been resolved, one cannot be purged. The exterior should be released first. After the exterior has been resolved when there is pain and obstruction in the lesser abdomen (xiao fu), it is possible to purge the stagnant blood. Tao He Cheng Qi Tang is appropriate.

2-35. 傷寒八九日 下之 胸滿煩驚 小便不利 譫語 一身盡重 不可轉側者 柴胡加龍骨牡 蠣湯主之. (107)

In Shang Han condition lasting eight to nine days, the purging method is applied, and there then occurs fullness in the chest, irritability, fright, urinary difficulty, delirious speech, heaviness, and inability to turn sides, Chai Hu Jia Long Gu Mu Li Tang governs.

2-36. 傷寒 脈浮 醫以火迫劫之 ^{亡陽} 必驚狂 臥起不安者 桂枝去芍藥加蜀漆牡蠣龍骨救 逆湯主之. (112)

When Shang Han condition with floating pulse is treated with fire methods, there will be fright, mania, and restlessness. Gui Zhi Qu Shao Yao Jia Shu Qi Mu Li Long Gu Jiu Ni Tang governs.

2-37. 燒針令其汗 針處被寒 核起而赤者 必發奔豚 ^{氣從少腹上衝心者} 灸其核上各一壯 與桂枝 加桂湯. (117)

A person who gets red swelling at the acupuncture point, caused by an attack of cold pathogens responding to fire needle induced sweating, will experience running piglet - the Qi surging upward from the lesser abdomen to the heart. This can be treated with a single unit of moxibustion on each swelling site and Gui Zhi Jia Gui Tang.

2-38. 火逆下之 因燒針煩燥者 桂枝甘草龍骨牡蠣湯主之. (118)

Gui Zhi Gan Cao Long Gu Mu Li Tang is indicated for irritability and nervousness after treatment with fire needle and purging methods.

2-39. 太陽病 過經 十餘日 心下溫溫欲吐 而胸中痛 大便反溏 腹微滿 鬱鬱微煩 先此時 自極吐下者 與調胃承氣湯 若不爾者 不可與 ○但欲嘔 胸 胃中痛 微 溏 弱者 此非柴胡湯證 以嘔故知極吐也・ (123)

In Tai Yang disorder that has lasted for over ten days, when there is epigastric stuffiness with a desire to vomit, chest pain, loose stool, mild fullness in the abdomen, and depression with mild irritability, and prior to these there occured extreme vomiting and diarrhea spontaneously, Tiao Wei Cheng Qi Tang can be applied. If there are no such symptoms, it cannot be used. A desire to vomit with pain in the chest and stomach and slightly loose stool is not a Chai Hu Tang pattern.

2-40. 太陽病六七日 表證仍在 脈微而沈 反不結胸 其人發狂者 以熱熱在下焦 小腹當硬 滿 小便自利者 下血乃愈 所以然者 以太陽隨經 證 瘀熱在裏故也 抵當湯主之. (124)

In Tai Yang disorder that has lasted for six to seven days, when there still exists exterior symptoms along with minute and deep pulse, but without obstruction in the chest (jie xiong), the person is manic due to heat accumulation in the lower burner. This situation can also be accompanied by hardness and fullness in the lesser abdomen and uninhibited urination, but recovery occurs once blood is expelled. This is because the pathogen of Tai Yang disorder penetrated other channels due to stagnant heat in the interior. Di Dang Tang governs.

2-41. 太陽病 身黃 脈沈結 小腹硬 小便不利者 爲無血也 小便自利 其人如狂者 血證諦也 抵當湯主之.(125)

Di Dang Tang is indicated for Tai Yang disorder with generalized jaundice, deep and knotted pulse, hardness in the lesser abdomen, uninhibited urination, and manic behavior. This is a blood pattern. However, if there is urinary difficulty, it is not a blood related pattern.

2-42. 傷寒有熱 少腹滿 應小便不利 今反利者 ^{爲有血也} 當可下之 ^{不可餘藥} 宜抵當丸.(126)

Di Dang Tang is appropriate to use when in Shang Han condition with heat, fullness in the lesser abdomen, usually with urinary difficulty. But lack of urinary difficulty indicates the condition is due to blood stagnation that should be purged.

太陽病結胸 (Chest Obstruction of Tai Yang Disorders)

病發於陽 而反下之 熱入 因作結胸 病發於陰 而反下之 因作痞也 所以成結胸者 以下之太早故也 結胸者 項亦強 如柔痙狀 下之則和 宜大陷胸丸. (131)

When the disease that stems from Yang is treated adversely by purging method, the heat enters the interior and causes chest obstruction(jie xiong). When the disease from yin is treated adversely by purgation, distension is generated. Chest obstruction is formed when purgation is applied too early, and is also accompanied by stiffness in the neck as in soft spasm. Da Xian Xiong Tang is appropriate to purge the stagnation.

3-1. 太陽病 脈浮而動數 ^{浮則爲風 數則爲熱 動則爲痛 數則爲虛} 頭痛發熱 微盜汗出 而反惡寒者 表未解也 醫反下之 動數變遲 脅內拒痛 短氣躁煩 心中懊憹 陽氣內陷 心下因硬 則爲結胸 大陷胸湯主之 ^{胃中空虛 客氣動膈} 若不大結胸 但頭汗出 餘處無汗 劑頸而還 小便不利 身必發黃也 宜大陷胸丸. (134)

Tai Yang disorder with floating, moving, and rapid pulse (floating means wind, rapid means heat, moving means pain, and rapid also means deficiency) and also with headache, fever, mild night sweating, and yet aversion to cold, means that the exterior has not been resolved. If a physician uses purging methods in adverse, the moving and rapid pulse will change to a slow pulse, and there will be pain in the ribcage, shortness of breath, agitation and irritability, anguish in the heart, and hardness below the heart due to internalized yang qi. This is called Jie Xiong -obstruction in the chest - and Da Xian Xiong Tang governs. If there is no chest obstruction but only sweating in the head not the rest of the body, and urinary difficulty, there will be generalized jaundice and Da Xian Xiong Wan is appropriate.

3-2. 傷寒六七日 結胸熱實 脈沈而緊 心下痛 按之石硬者 大陷胸湯主之. (135)

In Shang Han condition that has been present for six to seven days, when there is obstruction in the chest with excess heat, deep and tight pulse, epigastric pain, and hardness like stone below the heart on palpation, Da Xian Xiong Tang governs.

3-3. 傷寒十餘日 熱結在裏 復往來寒熱者 與大柴胡湯 但結胸無大熱 無大熱者 此爲水結在胸脅也 惟頭微汗出者 大陷胸湯主之. (136)

For Shang Han condition that has lasted for over ten days with heat obstruction in the interior and alternating chills and fever, give Da Chai Hu Tang. When there is only chest obstruction without a big fever, or mild sweating only in the head, the lack of fever indicates water obstruction in the chest and ribcage, and Da Xian Xiong Tang governs.

3-4. 太陽病 重發汗 而復下之 不大便 五 六日 舌上燥而渴 日晡所小有潮熱 發心胸大煩 從心下至小腹硬滿而痛 不可近者 大陷胸湯主之. (137)

When Tai Yang disorder has been treated by inducing sweating repeatedly and by repeated purgation, and there is no bowel movement for five to six days, dry tongue and thirst, mild tidal fever between 3pm and 5pm, severe irritability, and hardness, fullness, and pain from the epigastric area to the lesser abdomen that makes the person refuses to be palpated, Da Xian Xiong Tang governs.

少結胸者 正在心下 按之則痛 脈浮滑者 小陷胸湯主之. (138)

In minor chest obstruction, localized directly below the heart, where there is also pain on palpation, floating and slippery pulse, Xiao Xian Xiong Tang governs.

3-5. 病在陽 應以汗解之 反以冷水㇀之 若灌之 其熱被劫不得去 彌更益煩 肉上粟起 意欲飲水 反少渴者 服文蛤散. 若不差者 與五苓散. 寒實結胸 無熱證者 與三物小陷胸湯. 白散亦可服· (141)

When disease is in the yang level, it is appropriate to induce sweating to release the exterior. If it is adversely treated with cold water, the heat will appear to be suppressed but the cause won't actually be removed. Rather, it can become more severe, with irritability, skin problems like little bumps, a desire to drink water but little thirst. In this case, Wen Ge San can be given. If not completely resolved, give Wu Ling San. For chest obstruction due to cold excess, San Wu Xiao Xian Xiong Tang governs.

3-6. 婦人中風七八日續得寒熱 發作有時 經水適斷者 ^{此爲熱入血室} 其血必結 故使如瘧狀 發作有時 小柴胡湯主之. (144)

A Woman with Zhong Feng condition lasting seven to eight days, who gets periodic chills and fever, and amennorhea, these symptoms indicate that heat has entered the blood chamber. The blood will be stagnated, which lead to malaria-like symptom at regular intervals. Xiao Chai Hu Tang governs.

3-7. 傷寒六七日 發熱微惡寒 支節煩疼 微嘔 心下支結 外證未去者 柴胡桂枝湯主之. (146)

On the sixth to seventh day of Shang Han condition, when there is fever, mild aversion to cold, irritable pain of limb joints, mild nausea, and vertical prolonged congestion below the heart, Chai Hu Gui Zhi Tang governs, since the exterior has not been resolved yet.

3-8. 傷寒五六日 已發汗而復下之 胸脅滿微結 小便不利 渴而不嘔 但頭汗出 往來寒熱 心煩者 ^{此爲未解也} 柴胡桂枝乾薑湯主之. (147)

In Shang Han condition that has been present for five to six days that has been treated first with the sweating method and then with the purging method, and there presents fullness and mild obstruction in the chest and ribcage, urinary difficulty, thirst without nausea, sweating only in the head area, alternating chills and fever, and anxiety, all due to the condition not resolved yet, Chai Hu Gui Zhi Gan Jiang Tang governs.

3-9. 傷寒五六日 頭汗出 微惡寒 手足冷 心下滿 口不欲食 大便硬 脈細者 ^{此爲陽微結 必有表復 有裏也 脈沈 亦在裏也} ^{汗出爲陽微 假令純陰結 不得復有外證 悉入在裏 此爲半在裏半在外也 脈雖沈緊 不得爲少陰病 所以然者 少陰 不得有汗 今頭汗出 故知非少陰也} 可與小柴胡湯 設不了了者 得屎而解. (148)

In Shang Han condition that has been present for five to six days, when there is sweating in the head, mild averion to cold, cold hands and feet, fullness below the heart, loss of appetite, hard stools, and thready pulse, Xaio Chai Hu Tang can be applied. When the condition is not clearly resolved, the recovery will occur as soon as the stool passes. This all indicates mild yang obstruction. There will be exterior and interior conditions. The deep pulse means an interior condition. Sweating means mild yang. If pure yin is obstructed, there cannot be exterior symptoms since everything has entered the interior. This case, then, is half interior and half exterior, and it cannot be a Shao Yin disorder even if the pulse is deep and tight. There shouldn't be any sweating in Shao Yin disorder, but this case has sweating in the head. Therefore it is clear that this is not Shao Yin disorder.

3-10. 傷寒五六日 嘔而發熱者 柴胡湯證具 而以他藥下之 柴胡證仍在者 復與柴胡湯 ^此 ^{雖已下之 不爲逆也} 必蒸蒸而振 却發熱汗出而解 若心下滿而硬痛者 大陷胸湯主之 但滿 而不痛者 ^{此爲痞} 柴胡不中與之 宜半夏瀉心湯. (149)

Shang Han condition that has lasted for five to six days with nausea and fever is of Chai Hu Tang pattern. Even when it is treated with purging herbs, if the Chai Hu Tang signs are still present, Chai Hu Tang can still be used. This is not an adverse treatment although the purging method have already been applied. There will be steaming and shivering followed by fever and sweating with this formula, and the condition will be resolved. If there is fullness, hardness and pain below the heart, Da Xian Xiong Tang governs. If there is only fullness, but no pain (this is called Pi), Ban Xia Xie Xin Tang is appropriate, not Chai Hu.

3-11. 太陽中風 下利 嘔逆 ^{表解者 乃可攻之} 其人漐漐汗出 發作有時 頭痛 心下痞硬滿 引脅下痛 乾嘔 短氣 汗出 不惡寒者 ^{此表解 裏未和也} 十棗湯主之. (152)

In Zhong Feng condition of Tai Yang disorder with diarrhea and retching, when the exterior has resolved, the interior may still need to be treated. When the person has slight sweating at specific times, headache, epigastric distention, hardness and fullness, pulling hypochondriac pain, dry retching, shortness of breath, sweating without aversion to cold, it means that the exterior has resolved but the interior is not harmonized yet. Shi Zao Tang governs.

3-12. 太陽病 醫發汗 遂發熱惡寒 因復下之 心下痞 ^{表裏俱虛 陰陽氣竝竭} ^{無陽則陰獨} 復加燒針 因 胸煩 ^{面色清黃 膚瞤者 難治 今色微黃 手足溫者 易愈}. (153)

When Tai Yang disorder has been treated by inducing sweating and the person still has fever and chills, if the purging method is applied, there will be distention below the heart due to both interior and exterior deficiency, exhaustion of yin, yang, and qi, or no yang only yin. When the fire needling is added additionally, irritability in the chest occurs. If the complexion is bluish yellow with twitching skin, it is difficult to treat. But if the complexion is slightly yellow and the hands and feet are warm, it is easier to treat.

心下痞 按之濡 其脈關上浮者 大黃黃連瀉心湯主之. (154)

When there is distention below the heart that is soft upon palpation, and the pulse is floating on the guan position, Da Huang Huang Lian Xie Xin Tang governs.

心下痞 而復惡寒 汗出者 附子瀉心湯主之. (155)

When there is distention below the heart with relapsing chills and sweating, Fu Zi Xie Xin Tang governs.

心下痞 本以下之故 與瀉心湯 痞不解 其人渴而口燥煩 小便不利者 五苓散主之. (156)

When there is distention below the heart due to the application of the purging method, Xie Xin Tang can be used. If the epigastric distention is not relieved, and the person is thirsty with a dry mouth, irritability, and urinary difficulty, Wu Ling San governs.

3-13. 傷寒 汗出解之後 胃中不和 心下痞硬 乾噫 食臭 脅下有水氣 腹中雷鳴 下利者 生薑瀉心湯主之.(157)

In Shang Han condition, after the exterior is resolved by perspiration, but a person still gets indigestion, distention and hardness below the heart, dry belching with foul smells of food, hypochondriac water qi stasis, borborygmus, and diarrhea, Sheng Jiang Xie Xin Tang governs.

3-14. 傷寒中風 醫反下之 其人下利 日數十行 穀不化 腹中雷鳴 心下痞硬而滿 乾嘔 心煩不得安 醫見心下痞 謂病不盡 復下之 其痞益甚 此非結熱 但以胃中虛 客氣上逆 故使硬也 甘草瀉心湯主之. (158)

When Shang Han or Zhong Feng condition is adversely treated with the purging method, there will be diarrhea about ten times per day with undigested food, borborygmus, distention, hardness and fullness below the heart, dry retching, irritability, and uneasiness. If the physician mistakenly considers the congestion below the heart as the illness that has not resolved completely and applies purging again, the congestion will get worse. It is because these symptoms are not due to heat congestion but stomach deficiency with a counterflow of qi. Gan Cao Xie Xin Tang governs.

3-15. 傷寒服湯藥 下利不止 心下痞硬 服瀉心湯已 復以他藥下之 利不止 醫以理中與之 利益甚 理中者 理中焦 此利在下焦　赤石脂禹餘糧湯主之 復不止者 當利其小便. (159)

When Shang Han condition is treated with an herbal decoction and there is still incessant diarrhea and distention and hardness below the heart, and if Xie Xin Tang has already been applied and other purging formulas have been used, and the diarrhea will not stop or worsens even with Li Zhong Tang, it is because the Li Zhong Tang treats middle burner while this diarrhea is in the lower burner.

Chi Shi Zhi Yu Yu Liang Tang should be used, and if the diarrhea persists, urination should be promoted.

3-16. 傷寒發汗 若吐 若下 解後 心下痞硬 噫氣不除者 旋復代赭湯主之.(161)

Xuan Fu Da Zhe Tang is indicated for belching with epigastric distention and hardness even after the Shang Han condition is relieved by inducing sweating, vomiting or purging methods.

3-17. 太陽病 外證未除 而數下之 遂協熱而利 利下不止 心下痞硬 表裏不解者 桂枝人參湯主之. (163)

In Tai Yang disorder, when the exterior pattern is not resolved but the purging method has been applied several times, there will be fever accompanied by incessant diarrhea, distention and hardness below the heart, not to mention other unresolved exterior and interior symptoms. Gui Zhi Ren Shen Tang governs.

3-18. 傷寒大下後 復發汗 心下痞 惡寒者 表未解也 不可攻痞 當先解表 表解乃可攻痞. 解表 宜桂枝人參湯 攻痞宜大黃黃連瀉心湯 (164)

After the strong purging method is applied in Shang Han condition and sweating is induced again, a person may suffer distention below the heart and aversion to cold. This is due to an unresolved exterior where the distention cannot be cured. One should first resolve exterior, then can attack the distention once the exterior has been resolved. Gui Zhi Tang is appropriate to resolve the exterior and Da Huang Huang Lian Xie Xin Tang is appropriate to attack the distention.

3-19. 傷寒發熱 汗出不解 心中痞硬 嘔吐而下利者 大柴胡主之 (165)

When Shang Han condition with fever is not resolved with perspiration, and there is distention and hardness below the heart, nausea and vomiting, and diarrhea, Da Chai Hu Tang governs.

3-20. 傷寒 若吐 若下後 七八日不解 熱結在裏 表裏俱熱 時時惡風 大渴 舌上乾燥而煩 欲飲水數升者 白虎加人參湯主之. (168)

If Shang Han condition treated with vomiting or purging methods has not resolved in seven to eight days, and the heat is bound in interior with fever in both the exterior and interior, and there is occasional aversion to wind, severe thirst with dry tongue, irritability, and a desire to drink lots of water, Bai Hu Jia Ren Shen Tang governs.

3-21. 傷寒 無大熱 口燥渴 心煩 背微惡寒者 白虎加人參湯主之. (169)

Bai Hu Jia Ren Shen Tang is indicated for Shang Han condition without big fever but with dry mouth, thirst, irritability and a slight aversion to cold in the back.

3-22. 傷寒脈浮 發熱無汗 其表不解者 不可與白虎湯 渴欲飲水 無表證者 白虎加人參湯主之.(170)

Bai Hu Jia Ren Shen Tang governs Shang Han condition with a floating pulse, fever without sweating, thirst with a desire to drink water, but with no exterior pattern. If the exterior has not resolved, Bai Hu Tang cannot be used.

3-23. 太陽與少陽合病 自下利者 與黃芩湯 若嘔者 黃芩加半夏生薑湯主之.(172)

Huang Qin Tang can be applied to Tai Yang and Shao Yang combination disorder with spontaneous diarrhea. If nausea is also present, Huang Qin Jia Ban Xia Sheng Jiang Tang governs.

3-24. 傷寒 胸中有熱 胃中有邪氣 腹中痛 欲嘔吐者 黃連湯主之.(173)

Huang Lian Tang is indicated for Shang Han condition with fever in the chest, evil Qi in the stomach, pain in the abdomen, and a desire to vomit.

3-25. 傷寒八九日 風濕相搏 身體疼煩 不能自轉側 不嘔 不渴 脈浮虛而濇者 桂枝附子湯主之 若其人大便硬 小便不利者 去桂加白朮湯主之. (174)

When in Shang Han condition that has lasted eight to nine days with wind and dampness fighting each other, generalized bodyaches with irritability, inability to turn to the side, absence of nausea, absence of thirst, floating empty and choppy pulse, Gui Zhi Fu Zi Tang governs. If the person also has hard stool and urinary difficulty, Gui Zhi Qu Gui Jia Bai Zhu Tang.

3-26. 風濕相搏 骨節疼煩 ┌痛 不得屈伸 近之則痛劇 汗出短氣 小便不利 惡風不欲去衣 或身微腫者 甘草附子湯主之. (175)

When wind and dampness fight each other, and there is joint pain with irritability, pulling pain, an inability to bend or stretch, severe pain even with light touch, sweating, shortness of breath, urinary difficulty, an aversion to wind with no desire to undress, or occasional mild generalized edema, Gan Cao Fu Zi Tang governs.

3-27. 傷寒 脈浮滑 白虎湯主之. (176)

Bai Hu Tang is indicated for Shang Han condition with a floating and slippery pulse.

3-28. 傷寒 解而後 脈結代 心動悸 炙甘草湯主之. (177)

Zhi Gan Cao Tang should be applied when a pulse is knotted and intermittent with severe heart palpitations after the Shang Han condition has resolved.

辨陽明病 (Yang Ming Disorders)

4-1. 陽明之爲病 胃家實是也. (180)

Yang Ming disorder is characterized by an excess pattern of the stomach.

○ 問曰 陽明病外證云何. 答曰 身熱 汗自出 不惡寒 反惡熱也. (182)

The question is what are the outward symptoms of Yang Ming disorder. The answer is generalized fever, spontaneous sweating, no aversion to cold, but aversion to heat.

傷寒 發熱 無汗 嘔不能食 而反汗出┌┌然者 是轉屬陽明也. (185)

In Shang Han condition, when there is fever, absence of sweating, nausea with loss of appetite, if streaming sweat occurs, it means that the disorder has transformed to Yang Ming.

◯ 陽明病 不吐不下 心煩者 可與調胃承氣湯. (207)

In Yang Ming disorder, when neither vomiting nor purging method was applied, and there is irritability, Tiao Wei Cheng Qi Tang can be used.

4-2. 陽明病 脈遲 雖汗出 不惡寒者 其身必重 短氣 腹滿而喘 有潮熱 有潮熱者 此外欲解 可攻裏也 手足┌然汗出者 汗出者 此大便已硬也 大承氣湯主之. (208)

In Yang Ming disorder with slow pulse, when there is perspiration without aversion to cold, there will be generalized heaviness, shortness of breath, fullness in the abdomen, panting, tidal fever, and sweat streaming from hands and feet. Da Cheng Qi Tang should be applied, as the tidal fever indicates the exterior is about to resolve and one can attack the interior. In addition, sweating means the stool is already hard.

4-3. 陽明病 潮熱 大便微硬者 可與小承氣湯 不硬者 不可與之.

Xiao Cheng Qi Tang governs Yang Ming disorder with tidal fever and slightly hard stool. If it is not hard, this formula should not be given.

4-4. 傷寒若吐若下後不解 不大便五六日 以上 至十餘日 日晡所發潮熱 不惡寒 獨語如 見鬼狀. 若劇者 發則不識人 循衣摸牀 ┌惕而不安 微喘直視 脈弦者生 澀者死 微者 但發潮熱 譫語者 大承氣湯主之. 若一服利 則止後服 (212)

Shang Han condition that has not resolved after using vomiting or purging method may present an inability to defecate for more than five to six days, even up to ten days. Tidal fever in the late afternoon without aversion to cold may also be present, but with delirious speech and hallucinations. In severe cases, the person may not recognize others, may fiddle about with clothes and furniture, be easily frightened and restless, pant slightly, stare with glassy eyes, and speak deliriously. Da Cheng Qi Tang governs.

If the pulse is wiry, the person will live. If the pulse is choppy, the person will die. If the pulse is minute, there will be only tidal fever. If the person gets diarrhea after taking this formula, then stop taking it.

陽明病 譫語 發潮熱 脈滑而疾者 小承氣湯主之. (214)

Xiao Cheng Qi Tang is indicated for Yang Ming disorder with delirious speech, tidal fever, and slippery and racing pulse.

4-5. 三陽合病 腹滿身重 難以轉側 口不仁 面垢 譫語遺尿 發汗則譫語甚 下之則額上 生汗 手足逆冷 若自汗出者 白虎湯主之. (219)

In three Yang combination disorder, there is abdominal fullness, generalized heaviness, difficulty turning over, loss of taste, grimy complexion, delirious speech, and urinary incontinence. If sweating is induced, there will be delirious speech, and if the purging method is applied, there will be perspiration on the forehead and coldness in the hands and feet. If there is spontaneous sweating, Bai Hu Tang should be given.

4-6. 二陽俌病 太陽證罷 但發潮熱 手足┌┐汗出 大便難而譫語者 下之則愈 宜大承氣 湯. (220)

In the combination of two yang disorders, when Tai Yang symptoms are resolved and there is only tidal fever, streaming sweat from the hands and feet, difficult bowel movements, and delirious speech, the purging method will give immediate relief. Da Cheng Qi Tang is appropriate.

4-7. 陽明病 脈浮而緊 咽燥口苦 腹滿而喘 發熱汗出 不惡寒 反惡熱 身重. 若發汗則躁 心憒憒 反譫語. 若加溫鍼 必┌惕煩躁 不得眠. 若下之 則胃中空虛 客氣動膈 心 中懊┌ 舌上胎者 梔子豉湯主之.(221)

Yang Ming disorder can present a floating and tight pulse, dry throat and bitter taste in the mouth, abdominal fullness, panting, fever, sweating, aversion to heat (not aversion to cold), and generalized heaviness. If sweating is induced for this case, there will be restlessness, mental confusion, and delirious speech. If fire needle is applied, there will be irritability, restlessness and insomnia. If the purging method is applied, the stomach will become deficient and the evil Qi will attack the diaphragm, causing anguish in the heart along with a prominent coating on the tongue. Zhi Zi Chi Tang should be used.

若渴欲飲水 口乾舌燥者 白虎加人參湯主之. (222)

Bai Hu Jia Ren Shen Tang governs thirst with a desire to drink water, and also dry mouth and dry tongue.

若 脈微發熱 渴欲飲水 小便不利者 猪苓湯主之. (223)

Zhu Ling Tang is indicated for symptoms of thirst with a desire to drink water, urinary difficulty, and fever with floating pulse.

○ 陽明病 汗出多而渴者 不可與猪苓湯 以汗多胃中燥 猪苓湯復利其小便故也. (224)

Zhu Ling Tang is contraindicated in Yang Ming disorder with profuse sweating and thirst because the profuse sweating leads to dryness in the stomach and Zhu Ling Tang promotes urination.

4-8. 陽明病 下之 其外有熱 手足溫 不結胸 心中懊┌ 飢不能食 但頭汗出者 梔子豉湯主之. (228)

If Yang Ming disorder, treated by the purging method, presents exterior heat and warm hands and feet, it indicates that it is not chest obstruction (Jie Xiong). In addition to these symptoms, when there is anguish in the heart, hunger with inability to eat, and sweating only in the head, Zhi Zi Chi Tang governs.

4-9. 陽明病 發潮熱 大便溏 小便自可 胸脅滿不去者 小柴胡湯主之. (229)

Xiao Chai Hu Tang governs Yang Ming disorder with tidal fever, loose stools but normal urination, and persistent fullness in the chest and hypochondrium.

陽明病 脅下硬滿 不大便而嘔 舌上白胎者 可與小柴胡湯 上焦得通 津液得下 胃氣因和 身╒然汗出而解. (230)

Xiao Chai Hu Tang can be used for Yang Ming disorder with hypochondriac fullness and hardeness, constipation, nausea, and white coating on the tongue. When the upper burner is unblocked, body fluids will then descend, and the stomach qi will be harmonized. It will be resolved after generalized streaming sweat occurs.

4-10. 陽明病中風 脈弦浮大而短氣 腹都滿 脅下及心痛 久按之 氣不通 鼻乾不得汗 嗜臥 一身及面目悉黃 小便難 有潮熱 時時╒ 耳前後腫 刺之小差 外不解 病過十日 脈續浮者 與小柴胡湯. (231)

The symptoms of the Zhong Feng condition of Yang Ming disorder are wiry, floating and big pulse, shortness of breath, fullness in the whole abdomen, pain in the heart and hypochondrium, qi obstruction when pressure is applied for a long time, dry nose, inability to sweat, somnolence, jaundice in the eyes, face, and body, urinary difficulty, tidal fever, frequent hiccups, and swelling in front of and behind the ears. If the symptoms are slightly relieved by acupuncture, but the exterior is still not resolved after more than ten days, and the pulse is still floating, Xiao Chai Hu Tang should be applied.

脈但浮 無餘證者 與麻黃湯 _{若不尿 腹滿加╒者 不治} (232)

If there are no other symptoms besides a floating pulse, Ma Huang Tang can be applied. If the person cannot urinate and suffers from abdominal distention and incessant hiccups, there is no suggested treatment.

4-11. 陽明病 發熱汗出者 _{此爲熱越} 不能發黃也 但頭汗出 身無汗 劑頸而還 小便不利 渴引水漿者 _{此爲瘀熱在裏} 身必發黃 茵陳蒿湯主之. (236)

Yang Ming disorder with fever and sweating means that heat is dispersed and will not lead to jaundice. If sweating occurs only on the head and neck but not anywhere else, and there is also urinary difficulty and thirst with a tendency to drink fluids, it indicates heat stagnation in the interior, which will lead to generalized jaundice. Yin Chen Hao Tang governs.

4-12. 陽明證 其人喜忘者 必有蓄血 ^{所以然者 本有久瘀血 故令喜忘} 尿雖難 大便反易 而其色必黑者 宜抵當湯下之. (237)

When a person with the Yang Ming pattern is forgetful, there will be an accumulation of blood. This is due to a long standing stagnation of blood. If there is also hard stool but no difficulty in passing it, it will be black in color. It is appropriate to use Di Dang Tang to purge the blood stasis.

4-13. 陽明病 下之 心中懊ㄏ而煩 胃中有燥屎者 宜大承氣湯. ^{若有燥屎者 可攻 腹微渴滿 初頭硬 後必溏 者 不可攻之.} (238)

When, after treating Yang Ming disorder with the purging method, there is anguish in the heart, irritability, and dry stool, Da Cheng Qi Tang is appropriate. The attacking method can be used if there is dry stool. But if there is mild abdominal fullness, and a stool that is hard at the beginning and loose thereafter, the attacking method cannot.

4-14. 大下後 六七日不大便 煩不解 腹滿痛者 此有燥屎也 ^{所以然者 本有宿食故也} 宜大承氣湯. (241)

Da Cheng Qi Tang is recommended for cases where, after a strong purgation, there is no bowel movement for six to seven days, unresolved irritability, and abdominal fullness and pain due to dry stool (from undigested and stagnated food).

4-15. 食穀欲嘔者 屬陽明也 吳茱萸湯主之 ^{得湯反劇者 屬上焦也.} (243)

A desire to vomit after eating belongs to Yang Ming. Wu Zhu Yu Tang governs. If the symptoms gets more severe after taking this formula, it belongs to the Upper Burner.

4-16. 太陽病三日 發汗不解 蒸蒸發熱者 屬胃也 調胃承氣湯主之. (248)

After Tai Yang disorder lasting for three days, if the exterior is still not resolved with the sweating method and there is a persistent steaming fever, it means that this pattern belongs to the stomach. Tiao Wei Cheng Qi Tang governs.

4-17. 傷寒七八日 身黃如橘子色 小便不利 腹微滿者 茵陳蒿主之. (260)

In Shang Han condition that has lasted for seven to eight days, when there is generalized jaundice with an orange hue, urinary difficulty, and mild fullness in the abdomen, Yin Chen Hao Tang should be used.

4-18. 傷寒身黃發熱者 梔子蘗皮湯主之. (261)

Zhi Zi Bai Pi Tang is indicated for Shang Han condition with generalized jaundice and fever.

傷寒 瘀熱在裏 身必發黃 麻黃連軺赤小豆湯主之. (262)

Ma Huang Lian Qiao Chi Xiao Dou Tang is indicated for Shang Han condition with stagnated heat in the interior and generalized jaundice.

辨少陽病 (Shao Yang Disorders)

5-1. 少陽之爲病 口苦 咽乾 目眩也. (263)

The primary symptoms of Shao Yang disorder are bitter taste in the mouth, dry throat, and dizziness.

5-2. 本太陽病不解 轉入少陽者 脅下硬滿 乾嘔不能食 往來寒熱 尚未吐下 脈沈緊者 與 小柴胡湯. (266)

When Tai Yang disorder is unresolved and shifted into Shao Yang, there is hardness and fullness in the hypochondrium, dry retching, inability to eat, and alternating chills and fever. If neither vomiting nor purging methods have yet been applied, and the pulse is deep and tight, Xiao Chai Hu Tang is recommended.

5-3. 若已吐下 發汗 溫針 譫語 柴胡證罷 此爲壞病 知犯何逆 以法治之 (267)

If vomiting, purging, sweating, or warm needling have already been used and there is delirious speech, it indicates that the case has been treated adversely and is not the Chai Hu pattern anymore. One should find out what kind of adverse treatment was applied and give the appropriate treatment.

辨太陰病 (Tai Yin Disorders)

6-1. 太陰之爲病 腹滿而吐 食不下 自利益甚 時腹自痛 若下之 必胸下結硬. (273)

The primary symptoms of Tai Yin disorder are bloating in the abdomen, vomiting, inability to get food down, severe spontaneous diarrhea, and periodic spontaneous abdominal pain. If treated by the purging method, there will be congestion and hardeness below the chest.

太陰病 脈浮者 少可發汗 宜桂枝湯. (276)

In Tai Yin disorder with floating pulse, sweating can be induced. Therefore, Gui Zhi Tang is appropriate.

6-2. 本太陽病 醫反下之 因爾腹滿時痛者 屬太陰也 桂枝加芍藥湯主之. 大實痛者 桂枝加大黃湯主之. (279)

When Tai Yang disorder is adversely treated with the purging method and abdominal fullness with periodic pain results, it belongs to Tai Yin disorder and Gui Zhi Jia Shao Yao Tang governs. If there is extreme excess pain, Gui Zhi Jia Da Huang Tang governs.

辨少陰病 (Shao Yin Disorders)

7-1. 少陰之爲病 脈微細 但欲寐也. (281)

The primary symptoms of Shao Yin disorder are a minute and thready pulse and a desire only to sleep.

7-2. 少陰病 始得之 反發熱 脈沈者 麻黃細辛附子湯主之. (301)

When Shao Yin disorder has just started, but there is fever and a deep pulse, Ma Huang Xi Xin Fu Zi Tang should be applied.

7-3. 少陰病 得之二三日 麻黃附子甘草湯 微發汗. 以二三日無裏證 故微發汗也 (302)

Ma Huang Fu Zi Gan Cao Tang is indicated for Shao Yin disorder that has lasted for two to three days, to promote mild sweating. When there are no interior signs and symptoms on the second or third day, one can induce sweating gently.

7-4. 少陰病 得之二三日以上 心中煩 不得臥者 黃連阿膠湯主之. (303)

When in Shao Yin disorder that has lasted for more than two to three days there is irritability and inability to sleep, Huang Lian E Jiao Tang governs.

7-5. 少陰病 得之一二日 口中和 其背惡寒者 附子湯主之. (304)

Shao Yin disorder that has lasted one or two days with aversion to cold in the back and no thirst should be treated with Fu Zi Yang.

7-6. 少陰病 身體痛 手足寒 骨節痛 脈沈者 附子湯主之. (305)

Fu Zi Tang governs Shao Yin disorder with generalized body pain, cold extremities, joint pain, and deep pulse.

7-7. 少陰病 下利 便膿血者 桃花湯主之. (306)

Tao Hua Tang is indicated for Shao Yin disorder with diarrhea with pus and blood.

7-8. 少陰病 二三日至四 五日 腹痛 小便不利 下利不止 便膿血者 桃花湯主之. (307)

When in Shao Yin disorder that has lasted from two to three up to four to five days, there is abdominal pain, urinary difficulty, and incessant diarrhea with pus and blood, Tao Hua Tang governs.

7-9. 少陰病 吐利 手足逆冷 煩躁欲死者 吳茱萸湯主之. (309)

Wu Zhu Yu Tang governs Shao Yin disorder with vomiting, diarrhea, cold hands and feet, and irritability and agitation with suicidal impulses.

7-10. 少陰病 下利 咽痛 胸滿 心煩者 豬膚湯主之. (310)

Zhu Fu Tang is indicated for Shao Yin disorder with diarrhea, sore throat, fullness in the chest, and irritability.

7-11. 少陰病二三日 咽痛者 可與甘草湯 不差 與桔梗湯. (311)

A person with sore throat on a second or third day of Shao Yin disorder can be treated with Gan Cao Tang. If it is not resolved, Jie Geng Tang can be applied.

少陰病 咽中傷 生瘡 不能語言 聲不出者 半夏苦酒湯主之. (312)

Ban Xia Ku Jiu Tang should be used for Shao Yin disorder with sores and damage in the throat resulting in an inability to speak and a loss of voice.

少陰病 咽中痛 半夏散及湯主之. (313)

Ban Xia San Ji Tang is indicated for Shao Yin disorder with soreness in the throat.

7-12. 少陰病 下利 白通湯主之. (314)

Bai Tong Tang governs Shao Yin disorder with diarrhea.

7-13. 少陰病 下利 脈微者 與白通湯 利不止 厥逆無脈 乾嘔 煩者 白通加猪膽汁湯主之. (315)

Bai Tong Tang can be given for Shao Yin disorder with diarrhea and minute pulse. When there is incessant diarrhea, cold limbs, an absent pulse, retching, and irritability, Bai Tong jia Zhu Dan Zhi Tang governs.

7-14. 少陰病 二三日不已 至四五日 腹痛 小便不利 四肢沈重疼痛 自下利^{自下利者 此爲有水氣也} 其人或咳 或小便利 或下利 或嘔者 玄武湯主之. (317)

When in Shao Yin Disorder that has lasted four to five days, there is abdominal pain, urinary difficulty, heaviness and pain in the limbs, and diarrhea, it means there is water qi, and the person may cough, or have uninhibited urination, or diarrhea, or nausea, Zhen Wu Tang governs.

7-15. 少陰病 下利清穀 裏寒外熱 手足厥逆 脈微欲絶 身反不惡寒 其人面色赤 或腹痛 或乾嘔 或咽痛 或利止 脈不出者 通脈回逆湯主之. (317)

Tong Mai Si Ni Tang is indicated for Shao Yin disorder with interior cold and exterior heat signs and symptoms, including diarrhea containing undigested food, cold hands and feet, minute and dying out pulse, and absence of aversion to cold. The person may also have red complexion, abdominal pain, dry retching, sore throat, incessant diarrhea, or imperceptible pulse.

7-16. 少陰病 其人或咳 或悸 或小便不利 或腹中痛 或泄利下重者 回逆散主之. (318)

When in Shao Yin disorder the person has cough, heart palpitations, urinary difficulty, abdominal pain, or diarrhea with tenesmus, Si Ni San should be applied.

7-17. 少陰病 下利六 七日 咳而嘔渴 心煩不得眠者 猪苓湯主之. (319)

A person with Shao Yin disorder exhibiting diarrhea for six to seven days, cough, nausea, thirst, irritability, and inability to sleep should be treated with Zhu Ling Tang.

少陰病 得之二三日 口燥咽乾者 急下之 宜大承氣湯. (320)

In Shao Yin disorder that has lasted for two to three days, when there is dry mouth and throat, the purging method needs to be applied immediately. Da Cheng Qi Tang is appropriate.

7-18. 少陰病 自利清水 色純靑 心下必痛 口乾燥者 可下之 宜大承氣湯. (321)

Shao Yin disorder with watery greenish diarrhea, epigastric pain, and dry mouth can be treated with the purging method. Da Cheng Qi Tang is appropriate.

7-19. 少陰病 脈沈者 急溫之 宜回逆湯. (323)

Si Ni Tang is appropriate to rapidly warm the body for Shao Yin disorder with deep pulse.

7-20. 少陰病 飲食入口則吐 心中溫溫欲吐 復不能吐 始得之 手足寒 脈弦遲^{脈弦遲者 此胸中實} ^{當吐之} 不可下也. 若膈上有寒飮 乾嘔者 不可吐也 當溫之 宜回逆湯. (324)

Shao Yin disorder with vomiting after eating, oppression in the chest with nausea yet inability to vomit, cold hands and feet, and wiry and slow pulse indicating excess in the chest, cannot be treated with purging but should be treated with the vomiting method. If there is cold fluid above the diaphragm and dry retching, the vomiting method cannot be applied, but the warming method should be used with Si Ni Tang.

辨厥陰病 (Jue Yin Disorders)

8-1. 厥陰之爲病 消渴 氣上撞心 心中疼熱 飢而不欲食 食則 吐吐 下之 利不止. (326)

The primary manifestations of Jue Yin disorder are wasting and thirsting, qi surging upward to the heart, pain and heat in the heart, hunger with no desire to eat, vomiting of roundworms after eating, and incessant diarrhea if purging method is applied.

傷寒脈微而厥 至七八日 膚冷 其人躁 無暫安時者 此爲藏厥 非爲 厥也 厥者 其人當吐 令病者靜 而復時煩者 此爲藏寒 上入其膈 故煩 須更復止 得食而嘔 又煩 煩者 聞食臭出 其人當自吐 厥者 烏梅丸主之 又主久利. (338)

In Shang Han condition when there is a minute pulse and cold limbs lasting for seven to eight days, this person may also have cold skin, agitation and restlessness, this indicates visceral reversal, not roundworm reversal. In roundworm reversal, the person will vomit roundworms. In this case, the person is calm, but has periodic irritability which indicates visceral cold. When a patient gets irritable it may be due to roundworms ascending and entering the diaphragm. The irritability will eventually cease. When the person experiences nausea after eating and irritability, it is due to the roundworms smelling the malodor of food which can cause the person to spontaneously vomit roundworms. Wu Mei Wan governs for this round worm reversal, as well as longstanding diarrhea.

8-2. 傷寒脈滑 而厥者 裏有熱也 白虎湯主之. (350)

Bai Hu Tang is indicated for Shang Han condition presented by slippery pulse and the coldness of the limbs due to interior heat.

8-3. 手足厥寒 脈細欲絶者 當歸回逆湯主之. (351)

Dang Gui Si Ni Tang should be used for a person with coldness of the limbs and minute and dying out pulse.

8-4. 若其人內有久寒者 宜當歸回逆加吳茱萸生薑湯. (352)

If the person has enduring cold on the interior, Dang Gui Si Ni Jia Wu Zhu Yu Sheng Jiang Tang is appropriate.

○ 大汗出熱不去 內拘急 四肢疼 又下利 厥逆而惡寒者 回逆湯主之. (353)

A person with severe sweating, prolonged fever, abdominal spasms, pain in the limbs, diarrhea, coldness in the limbs, and aversion to cold should be treated with Si Ni Tang.

大汗 若大下利 而厥冷者 回逆湯主之. (354)

Si Ni Tang is indicated for a person with severe perspiration, severe diarrhea, and coldness in the limbs.

病人手足厥冷 脈乍緊 邪結在胸中 心下滿而煩 飢不能食者 病在胸中 當須吐之 宜瓜蒂散. (355)

Coldness in the limbs and a tight pulse indicate that the evil is obstructed in the chest. Epigastric fullness, irritability, and hunger with inability to eat indicate that the disease is in the chest. The person should be treated by the vomiting method with Gua Di San.

傷寒 厥而心下悸者 宜先治水 當服茯苓甘草湯 却治其厥 不爾 水漬入胃 必作利也. (356)

When the Shang Han condition is accompanied by coldness of the limbs and palpitation below the heart, it is appropriate to treat the water first. Fu Ling Gan Cao Tang should be applied, then the coldness of the limbs can also be treated. If not treated in this way, the water will enter the stomach resulting in diarrhea.

傷寒六七日 大下後 寸脈沈而遲 手足厥逆 與回逆湯 下部脈不至 咽喉不利 唾膿血 泄利 不止者 為難治 屬麻黃升麻湯. (357)

When the Shang Han condition has lasted for six to seven days and after strong pulging method has been applied, if the Cun pulse is deep and slow and there is coldness of the limbs, give Si Ni Tang. When the Chi pulse fails to arrive normally and there is a discomfort in the throat, spitting of pus and blood, and incessant diarrhea, it is hard to treat. In this case, Ma Huang Sheng Ma Tang governs.

8-5. 傷寒 本自寒下 醫復吐下之 寒格 更逆吐下 若食入口即吐 乾薑黃芩黃連人參湯主
之. (359)

Shang Han condition originally with spontaneous cold diarrhea that has been mistreated with an emetic or purgative will result in mutual repulsion between upper jiao heat and lower jiao cold. If it is mistreated with emetic and purgative again and the person vomits after eating food, Gan Jiang Huang Qin Huang Lian Ren Shen Tang should be applied.

下利清穀 裏寒外熱 汗出而厥者 通脈回逆湯主之. (370)

Tong Mai Si Ni Tang is indicated for diarrhea with undigested food, interior cold and exterior heat, sweating, and coldness in the limbs.

熱利下重者 白頭翁湯主之. (371)

Bai Tou Weng Tang should be used for heat diarrhea with tenesmus.

○ 下利 腹脹滿 身體疼痛者 先溫其裏 乃攻其表 溫裏宜回逆湯 攻表宜桂枝湯. (372)

When there is diarrhea, abdominal distention and fullness and generalized pain, first warm the interior, then attack the exterior. Si Ni Tang is appropriate to warm the interior and Gui Zhi Tang is appropriate to attack the exterior.

○ 下利 欲飲水者 以有熱故也 白頭翁湯主之. (373)

Diarrhea with a desire to drink water indicates that it is due to heat. Bai Tou Weng Tang governs.

○ 下利 譫語者 有燥屎也 宜小承氣湯. (374)

Diarrhea with delirious speech indicates that there is dry stool. Xiao Cheng Qi Tang is appropriate.

Angie Kim, Ph.D., L.Ac.

○ 下利後 更煩 按之心下濡者 爲虛煩也 宜梔子豉湯. (375)

After diarrhea, if a person gets more irritable and the epigastric area is soft on palpation, it indicates deficient type of irritability. Zhi Zi Chi Tang is appropriate.

○ 乾嘔 吐涎沫 頭痛者 吳茱萸湯主之. (378)

Wu Zhu Yu Tang is indicated for dry retching, vomiting of foamy saliva, and headache.

辨厥陰病霍亂 (Jue Yin Disorders with Huo Luan)

○ 問曰 病有霍亂何 答曰 嘔吐而利 此名霍亂. (382)

Question: What is the disease of Huo Luan? Answer: Vomiting and Diarrhea is called Huo Luan.

○ 問曰 病發熱頭痛 身疼惡寒 吐利者 此屬何病 答曰 此名霍亂 霍亂自吐下 又利止 復更發熱也. (383)

Question: What is the name of the disease when there is headache with fever, generalized pain, vomiting, and diarrhea? Answer. That is called Huo Luan. In Huo Luan, there is spontaneous vomiting and diarrhea, the diarrhea stops, and there will be a fever again.

9-1. 吐利惡寒 脈微而復利 利止 亡血也 回逆加人參湯主之. (385)

Si Ni Jia Ren Shen Tang should be used when there is vomiting, diarrhea, aversion to cold, a minute pulse, and blood collapse when the diarrhea stops.

9-2. 吐利霍亂 頭痛發熱 身疼痛 熱多欲飲水者 五苓散主之 寒多不用水者 理中丸主之. (386)

Wu Ling San governs when in Huo Luan, there is vomiting, diarrhea, headaches, fever, generalized pain, and a desire to drink water due to dominant heat. Li Zhong Wan is indicated for patients with absence of thirst due to dominant cold.

9-3. 吐利汗出 發熱惡寒 四肢拘急 手足厥冷者 回逆湯主之. (388)

Si Ni Tang is indicated for cases with vomiting, diarrhea, sweating, fever, aversion to cold, spasms of the limbs, and coldness of the hands and feet.

9-4. 旣吐且利 小便復利 而大汗出 下利清穀 內寒外熱 脈微欲絶者 回逆湯主之. (389)

Si Ni Tang should be used when there is vomiting, diarrhea with undigested food, polyuria, excessive sweating, a minute and dying out pulse, and interior cold with exterior heat.

9-5. 吐已下斷 汗出而厥 四肢拘急不解 脈微欲絶者 通脈回逆加猪膽汁湯主之. (390)

Tong Mai Si Ni Jia Zhu Dan Zhi Tang governs when vomiting and diarrhea have ceased, but there is sweating, cold extremities, spasms of the limbs, and a minute and dying out pulse.

辨陰陽易差後勞復病 (Yin Yang Exchange and Taxation Relapses)

傷寒陰陽易之爲病 其人身體重 少氣 少腹裏急 或引陰中拘攣 熱上衝胸 頭重不欲擧 眼中生花 膝脛拘急者 燒褌散主之. (392)

In Shang Han condition with yin yang exchange disease, when the person has generalized heaviness, shortage of qi, lesser abdominal spasm, or spasms in genitals, heat surging up to the chest, heaviness in the head with no desire to lift it, visual disturbances, and spasms of the knees and lower leg, Shao Kun San governs.

10-1. 大病差後 勞復者 枳實梔子豉湯主之. (393)

Zhi Shi Zhi Zi Chi Tang should be used when there is relapse due to excessive physical and mental stress after a major illness is cured.

10-2. 傷寒差以後 更發熱 小柴胡湯主之. 脈浮者 少以汗解之 脈沈實者 少以下解之. (394)

Xiao Chai Hu Tang is indicated for relapses of fever after Shang Han condition is cured. If the pulse is floating, it is appropriate to induce mild sweating, and if the pulse is deep and excess, mild purging will resolve the disease.

10-3. 大病差後 從腰以下有水氣者 牡蠣澤瀉散主之. (395)

Mu Li Ze Xie San should be applied to a person with edema below the waist after a major disease is cured.

10-4. 大病差後 喜唾 久不了了 胸上有寒 當以丸藥溫之 宜理中丸. (396)

Li Zhong Wan is recommended after a major disease is cured, when there is continued expectoration of sputum due to coldness above the chest.

10-5. 傷寒解後 虛羸少氣 逆欲吐 竹葉石膏湯主之. (397)

Zhu Ye Shi Gao Tang should be used after Shang Han condition is resolved, when there is weakness, emaciation, shortage of qi, and counterflow of qi with a desire to vomit.

Chapter 5

Conclusion

In the history of Traditional Asian Medicine, various diagnostic systems and methods have been developed. In this book, the theories and the clinical applications are described in a way that both common and individual physiology and pathology are taken into consideration. To summarize the procedure of this diagnostic approach, it can be explained roughly with these five virtual steps as below.

First, determine what kind of constitution your patient is. As described in Chapter 1, constitutional diagnosis should be made comprehensively based on all three of the appearances, the nature of the disposition, and the pathological symptoms. Among modern studies in an effort to improve the stability of diagnosis, the studies on voice characteristics for each constitution and the studies on the Sasang Constitutional Body Trunk Measurement are valuable.

Diagnosis using voice is one of the important parts in SCM. The relation between SC types and voice is referred in the literatures. Taiyangs's voice is resonant, clear, and loud. It was derived from good respiratory organs. Tai Yin types have a raspy baritone voice, which sounds thick, heavy, and grave. Shao Yang types have clear, fast, and high-pitched voice. They are talkative, hasty, and vigorous. Shao Yin type's voice is calm and easy. It sounds gentle, slow, and lively.[37]

Although the diagnosis based on the Sasang Constitutional Body Trunk Measurement is not completely reliable, it is useful to keep in mind that the peson with prominently expanded waist line most likely has a hyperactive liver.

---

[37] Jun-Su Jang, Young-Su Kim, Boncho Ku, and Jong Yeol Kim,<Recent Progress in Voice-Based Sasang Constitutional Medicine: Improving Stability of Diagnosis>

Second, identify whether this person has interior condition or exterior pattern. The differentiation of interior and exterior pattern based on each constitution is described in the table as below.

	Exterior pattern	Interior pattern
Shao Yin	Exterior Excess syndrome (chills and fever, no sweating) Exterior Deficiency Syndrome (Collapsed Yang in SCM) (chills and fever, sweating)	Tai Yin Syndrome (digestive problem without thirst or bodyache) Shao Yin Syndrome (digestive problem with thirst and an abnormal sensation of the mouth, bodyache)
Shao Yang	Shaoyang Wind Attack Syndrome (bitter taste in the mouth, dry throat, dizziness, tinnitus, congestion in the chest, alternating chills and fever) Collapsed Yin Syndrome (Mang Yin) (mainly with diarrhea)	Excess Yang Syndrome (excess heat in the chest and diaphragm, mainly with constipation) Deficient Yin Syndrome (with empty heat)
Tai Yin	Exterior cold Cold Syndrome in the epigastrium	Dry heat syndrome Yin Blood Exhaustion Syndrome
Tai Yang	Jieyi (解㑊) Syndrome (weakness in the lower body)	Yege(噎膈) or Fanwei(反胃) (disphasia or vomiting)

Third, identify whether this person has heat pattern or cold pattern. Although the treatment principle for Shaoyins is mainly to fortify yang of spleen and kidneys, the cooling herbs can still be administered in addition to qi or yang tonic herbs when there is heat pattern present in their condition, and vice versa for Shaoyangs.

Forth, identify which channel disorder does his or her condition belong to among six channel disorders of Shang Han Lun. To implement this step, it is important to understand the primary symptoms of each channel disorder inside and out.

In Tai Yang Disorder, the pulse is floating, the head and neck are stiff and painful, and there is aversion to cold. Yang Ming disorder is characterized by an excess pattern of the stomach. The primary symptoms of Shao Yang disorder are bitter taste in the mouth, dry throat, and dizziness.

The primary symptoms of Tai Yin disorder are bloating in the abdomen, vomiting, inability to get food down, severe spontaneous diarrhea, and periodic spontaneous abdominal pain. If treated by the purging method, there will be congestion and hardeness below the chest. The primary symptoms of Shao Yin disorder are a minute and thread pulse and a desire only to sleep. The primary manifestations of Jue Yin disorder are wasting and thirsting, qi surging upward to the heart, pain and heat in the heart, hunger with no desire to eat, vomiting of roundworms after eating, and incessant diarrhea if purging method is applied.

Fifth, identify the signs and symptoms of the disorder that is meaningful in clinical diagnosis, and choose an herbal formula based on the indication of herbs, formulas and/or the context of Shang Han Lun. The modern interpretations of Shang Han Lun based on clinical practice need to be shared among contemporary practitioners.

Appendix

Classical Formulas with Ingredients

Gui Zhi Formula Family

Gui Zhi Tang: Gui Zhi 6, Shao Yao 6, Sheng Jiang 6, Da Zao 6, Gan Cao 4

Gui Zhi Jia Gui Tang: Gui Zhi Tang + Gui Zhi 4

Gui Zhi Jia Shao Yao Tang: Gui Zhi Tang + Shao Yao 6

Gui Zhi Qu Shao Yao Tang: Gui Zhi Tang – Shao Yao 6

Gui Zhi Jia Ge Gen Tang: Gui Zhi Tang + Ge Gen 8

Gua Lou Gui Zhi Tang: Gui Zhi Tang + Gua Lou Gen 4

Gui Zhi Jia Huang Qi Tang: Gui Zhi Tang + Huang Qi 4

Gui Zhi Jia Shao Yao Da Huang Tang: Gui Zhi Tang + Shao Yao 6, Da Huang 2

Gui Zhi Jia Hou Po Xing Zi Tang: Gui Zhi Tang + Hou Po 4, Xing Ren 4

Wu Tou Gui Zhi Tang: Gui Zhi Tang + Da Wu Tou Jian (Wu Tou 10, honey 16)

Gui Zhi Jia Fu Zi Tang: Gui Zhi Tang + Fu Zi 2 or 3

Gui Zhi Jia Zhu Fu Tang: Gui Zhi Tang + Zhu 6, Fu Zi 2 or 3

Gui Zhi Jia Ling Zhu Fu Tang: Gui Zhi Jia Zhu Fu Tang + Fu Ling 6

Gui Zhi Qu Shao Yao Jia Fu Zi Tang: Gui Zhi Qu Shao YaoTang + Fu Zi 2 or 3

Gui Zhi Fu Zi Tang: Fu Zi 6~9, Gui Zhi 8, Sheng Jiang 6, Da Zao 6, Gan Cao 4

Bai Zhu Fu Zi Tang (Gui Zhi Fu Zi Qu Gui Jia Zhu Tang): Fu Zi 6~9, Sheng Jiang 6, Da Zao 6, Gan Cao 4

Gui Zhi Qu Gui Jia Ling Zhu Tang: Gui Zhi Tang – Gui Zhi 6 + Fu Ling 6, Zhu 6

Gui Gang Zao Cao Huang Xin Fu Tang: Gui Zhi Qu Shao Yao Tang + Ma Huang Fu Zi Xi Xin Tang

Gui Zhi Jia Long Gu Mu Li Tang: Gui Zhi Tang + Long Gu 6, Mu Li 6

Gui Zhi Qu Shao Yao Jia Shu Qi Long Gu Mu Li Jiu Ni Tang: Gui Zhi Qu Shao Yao Tang + Mu Li 10, Long Gu 8, Shu Qi 6

Gui Zhi Jia Shao Yao Sheng Jiang Ge Yi Liang Ren Shen San Liang Xin Jia Tang: Gui Zhi Tang + Shao Yao 2, Sheng Jiang 2, Ren Shen 6

Gui Zhi Er Ma Huang Yi Tang: Gui Zhi 5.4, Shao Yao 4, Sheng Jiang 4, Da Zao 4, Gan Cao 3.4, Ma Huang 2, Xing Ren 2

Gui Zhi Er Yue Bi Yi Tang: Da Zao 7.4, Sheng Jiang 6, Shi Gao 5.4, Gui Zhi 4, Shao Yao 4, Ma Huang 4, Gan Cao 4

Gui Zhi Ma Huang Ge Ban Tang: Gui Zhi 5, Shao Yao 3, Sheng Jiang 3, Da Zao 3, Gan Cao 3, Ma Huang 3, Xing Ren 3

Xiao Jian Zhong Tang: Yi Tang 32, Shao Yao12, Gui Zhi 6, Sheng Jiang 6, Da Zao 6, Gan Cao 6

Fu Ling Jian Zhong Tang: Xiao Jian Zhong Tang + Fu Ling 6

Huang Qi Jian Zhong Tang: Xiao Jian Zhong Tang + Huang Qi 3

Huang Qi Gui Zhi Wu Wu Tang: Sheng Jiang 12, Huang Qi 6, Shao Yao 6, Gui Zhi 6, Da Zao 6

Huang Qi Shao Yao Gui Zhi Ku Jiu Tang: Huang Qi 10, Shao Yao 6, Gui Zhi 6, Ku Jiu 40ml

Gui Zhi Gan Cao Tang: Gui Zhi 24, Gan Cao 12

Ban Xia San Ji Tang: Ban Xia 6, Gui Zhi 6, Gan Cao 6

Gan Cao Fu Zi Tang: Gui Zhi 8, Fu Zi 4~6, Zhu 4, Gan Cao 4

Gui Zhi Gan Cao Long Gu Mu Li Tang: Gui Zhi 6, Gan Cao 6, Long Gu 6, Mu Li 6

Gui Zhi Ren Shen Tang: Gui Zhi 8, Gan Cao 8, Zhu 6, Ren Shen 6, Gan Jiang 6

Gui Zhi Fu Ling Wan: Gui Zhi 6, Fu Ling 6, Mu Dan Pi 6, Tao Ren 6, Shao Yao 6

Fu Ling Formula Family

Fu Ling Gan Cao Tang: Fu Ling 6, Sheng Jiang 6, Gui Zhi 4, Gan Cao 2

Fu Ling Xing Ren Gan Cao Tang: Fu Ling 6, Xing Ren 4, Gan Cao 2

Kui Zi Fu Ling San: Kui Zi 6, Fu Ling 6

Ling Jiang Zhu Gan Tang: Fu Ling 8, Gan Jiang 8, Zhu 4, Gan Cao 4

Ling Gui Zhu Gan Tang: Fu Ling 8, Gui Zhi 6, Zhu 4, Gan Cao 4

Ling Gui Gan Zao Tang: Fu Ling 16, Gui Zhi 8, Da Zao 8, Gan Cao 6

Ling Gui Wei Gan Tang: Fu Ling 8, Gui Zhi 8, Wu Wei Zi 6, Gan Cao 6

Ling Gan Wu Wei Jiang Xin Tang: Fu Ling 8, Gan Cao 6, Wu Wei Zi 6, Gan Jiang 6, Xi Xin 6

Ling Gan Jiang Wei Xin Xia Tang: Ling Gan Wu Wei Jiang Xin Tang + Ban Xia 12

Ling Gan Jiang Wei Xin Xia Ren Tang: Ling Gan Jiang Wei Xin Xia Tang + Xing Ren 6

Ling Gan Jiang Wei Xin Xia Ren Huang Tang: Ling Gan Jiang Wei Xin Xia Ren Tang + Da Huang 6

Fu Ling Ze Xie Tang: Fu Ling 16, Ze Xie 8, Sheng Jiang 8, Zhu 6, Gui Zhi 4, Gan Cao 4

Ze Xie Tang: Ze Xie 15, Zhu 6

Wu Ling San: Ze Xie 10, Zhu Ling 6, Zhu 6, Fu Ling 6, Gui Zhi 4

Yin Chen Wu Ling San: Yin Chen Hao 32, Ze Xie 5, Zhu Ling 3, Zhu 3, Fu Ling 3, Gui Zhi 2

Zhu Ling Tang: Fu Ling 6, Zhu Ling 6, Ze Xie 6, Hua Shi 6, E Jia 6

Zhu Ling San: Zhu Ling 6, Fu Ling 6, Zhu 6

Mu Li Ze Xie San: Mu Li 6, Ze Xie 6, Gua Lou Gen 6, Shu Qi 6, Ting Li 6, Shang Lu Gen 6, Hai Zao 6

Ba Wei Wan: Gan Di Huang 16, Shan Yao 8, Shan Zhu Yu 8, Ze Xie 6, Fu Ling 6, Mu Dan Pi 6, Gui Zhi 4, Fu Zi 4

Gua Lou Qu Mai Wan: Fu Ling 6, Shan Yao 6, Gua Lou Gen 4, Fu Zi 2~3, Qu Mai 2

Ma Huang Formula Family

Ma Huang Tang: Ma Huang 6, Xing Ren 6, Gui Zhi 4, Gan Cao 2

Ma Huang Jia Zhu Tang: Ma Huang Tang + Zhu 8

Ma Huang Jia Zhu Fu Tang: Ma Huang Jia Zhu Tang + Fu Zi 3

Ma Huang Gan Cao Tang: Ma Huang 8, Gan Cao 4

Ma Huang Fu Zi Gan Cao Tang: Ma Huang 4, Gan Cao 4, Fu Zi 2~3

Ma Huang Fu Zi Tang: Ma Hung 6, Gan Cao 4, Fu Zi 2~3

Ma Huang Fu Zi Xi Xin Tang: Ma Huang 4, Xi Xin 4, Fu Zi 2~3

Ma Xing Gan Shi Tang: Shi Gao 24, Ma Huang 12, Xing Ren 6, Gan Cao 6

Ma Xing Yi Gan Tang: Yi Yi Ren 24, Ma Huang 12, Xing Ren6, Gan Cao 6

Mu Li Tang: Mu Li 12, Ma Huang 12, Shu Qi 9, Gan Cao 6

Ban Xia Ma Huang Wan: Ban Xia, Ma Huang, Half and Half with honey

Xiao Qing Long Tang: Ban Xia 12, Ma Huang 6, Shao Yao 6, Wu Wei Zi 6, Gan Jiang 6, Gan Cao 6, Gui Zhi 6, Xi Xin 6

Da Qing Long Tang: Shi Gao 16, Ma Huang 12, Sheng Jiang 6, Da Zao 6, Gui Zhi 4, Gan Cao 4, Xing Ren 4

Wen Ge Tang: Wen Ge 10, Shi Gao 10, Ma Huang 6, Sheng Jiang 6, Da Zao 6, Gan Cao 6, Xing Ren 4

Yue Bi Tang: Shi Gao 16, Ma Huang 12, Da Za 8, Sheng Jiang 6, Gan Cao 4

Yue Bi Jia Zhu Tang: Yue Bi Tang + Zhu 8

Yue Bi Jia Ban Xia Tang: Yue Bi Tang + Ban Xia 12

Ge Gen Formula Family

Ge Gen Tang: Ge Gen 8, Ma Huang 6, Sheng Jiang 6, Da Zao 6, Gui Zhi 4, Shao Yao 4, Gan Cao 4

Ge Gen Jia Jie Geng Tang: Ge Gen Tang + Jie Geng 6

Ge Gen Jia Da Huang Tang: Ge Gen Tang + Da Huang 2~6

Ge Gen Jia Zhu Fu Tang: Ge Gen Tang + Zhu 6, Fu Zi 2~6

Ge Gen Jia Ban Xia Tang: Ge Gen Tang + Ban Xia 12

Ge Gen Huang Qin Huang Lin Tang: Ge Gen 24, Huang Qin 9, Huang Lian 9, Gan Cao 6

Chai Hu Formula Family

Xiao Chai Hu Tang: Chai Hu 16, Ban Xia 12, Huang Qin 6, Ren Shen 6, Sheng Jiang 6, Da Zao 6, Gan Cao 6

Chai Hu Jia Gui Zhi Tang: Xiao Chai Hu Tang + Gui Zhi 6

Chai Hu Jia Mang Xiao Tang: Xiao Chai Hu Tang + Mang Xiao 8~12

Chai Hu Qu Ban Xia Jia Gua Lou Tang: Xiao Chai Hu Tang − Ban Xia 12 + Gua Lou Gen 8

Chai Hu Gui Zhi Tang: Chai Hu 8, Ban Xia 6, Gui Zhi 3, Shao Yao 3, Sheng Jiang 3, Ren Shen 3, Da Zao 3, Huang Qin 3, Gan Cao 2

Chai Hu Gui Zhi Gan Jiang Tang: Chai Hu 16, Gua Lou Gen 8, Huang Qin 6, Gui Zhi 6, Gan Jiang 4, Mu Li 4, Gan Cao 4

Chai Hu Jia Long Gu Mu Li Tang: Chai Hu 8, Ban Xia 6, Da Huang 4, Huang Qin 3, Long Gu 3, Mu Li 3, Gui Zhi 3, Fu Ling 3, Sheng Jiang 3, Da Zao 3, Ren Shen 3

Da Chai Hu Tang: Chai Hu 16, Ban Xia 12, Sheng Jiang 10, Zhi Shi 8, Huang Qin 6, Shao Yao 6, Da Zao 6, Da Huang 4

Da Chai Hu Jia Mang Xiao Tang: Da Chai Hu Tang + Mang Xiao 8~12

Shi Gao Formula Family

Bai Hu Tang: Shi Gao 32, Geng Mi 25, Zhi Mu 12, Gan Cao 4

Bai Hu Jia Ren Shen Tang: Shi Gao 32, Geng Mi 26, Zhi Mu 12, Ren Shen 6, Gan Cao 4

Bai Hu Jia Gui Zhi Tang: Shi Gao 32, Geng Mi 26, Zhi Mu 12, Gui Zhi 6, Gan Cao 4

Zhu Ru Shi Gao Tang: Shi Gao 32, Mai Men Dong 20, Geng Mi 20, Ban Xia 12, Ren Shen 6, Zhu Ru 6, Gan Cao 4

Da Huang / Mang Xiao Formula Family

Xiao Cheng Qi Tang: Da Huang 12, Zhi Shi 9, Hou Po 6

Hou Po San Wu Tang: Hou Po 16, Zhi Shi 10, Da Huang 8

Hou Po Qi Wu Tang: Hou Po 16, Zhi Shi 10, Sheng Jiang 10, Da Huang 6, Gan Cao 6, Da Zao 5, Gui Zhi 4

Da Cheng Qi Tang: Hou Po 16, Mang Xiao 12, Zhi Shi 10, Da Huang 8

Da Huang Huang Lian Xie Xin Tang: Da Huang 6, Huang Lian 3

Xie Xin Tang: Da Huang 12, Huang Qin 6, Huang Lian 6

Fu Zi Xie Xin Tang: Da Huang 6, Fu Zi 3~4.5, Huang Qin 3, Huang Lian 3

Da Huang Fu Zi Tang: Fu Zi 6~9, Da Huang 6, Xi Xin 4

Da Huang Gan Sui Tang: Da Hunag 8, E Jiao 4, Gan Sui 4

Di Dang Tang: Da Huang 6, Shui Zhi 4, Meng Chong 4, Tao Ren 2

Ju Pi Da Huang Po Xiao Tang: Da Huang 12, Mang Xiao 12, Ju Pi 6

Da Huang Xiao Shi Tang: Da Huang 8, Huang Bai 8, Xiao Shi 8, Zhi Zi 4

Da Huang Mu Dan Pi Tang: Gua Zi 20, Da Huang 8, Mu Dan Pi 6, Mang Xiao 4, Tao Ren 4

Da Huang Gan Cao Tang: Da Huang 12, Gan Cao 6

Tiao Wei Cheng Qi Tang: Da Huang 8, Mang Xiao 4, Gan Cao 4

Tao He Cheng Qi Tang: Da Huang 8, Tao Ren 4, Gui Zhi 4, Gan Cao 4, Mang Xiao 4

Da Xian Xiong Tang: Da Huang 16, Mang Xiao 10, Gan Sui 2

Da Xian Xiong Wan: Mang Xiao 20, Da Huang 16, Xing Ren 12, Ting Li 10, Gan Sui powder 2, honey 32

Gan Cao Formula Family

Gan Cao Tang: Gan Cao 6

Jie Geng Tang: Jie Geng 6, Gan Cao 6

Pai Nong Tang: Jie Geng 9, Da Zao 7.5, Gan Cao 6, Sheng Jiang 3

Shao Yao Gan Cao Tang: Shao Yao 12, Gan Cao 12

Gan Sui Ban Xia Tang: Ban Xia 12, Gan Cao 12, Shao Yao 6, Gan Sui 2~6, honey 16

Shao Yao Gan Cao Fu Zi Tang: Shao Yao 9, Gan Cao 9, Fu Zi 3~4.5

Gan Mai Da Zao Tang: Xiao Mai 32, Gan Cao 6, Da Zao 5

Sheng Jiang Gan Cao Tang: Sheng Jiang 10, Gan Cao 8, Da Zao 7.5, Ren Shen 6

Gan Cao Gan Jiang Tang: Gan Cao 12, Gan Jiang 6

Fu Zi Formula Family

Si Ni Tang: Gan Cao 6, Gan Jiang 4.5, Fu Zi 3~4.5

Tong Mai Si Ni Tang: Gan Jiang 9, Gan Cao 6, Fu Zi 3~4.5

Si Ni Jia Ren Shen Tang: Si Ni Tang + Ren Shen 3

Fu Ling Si Ni Tang: Fu Ling 12, Gan Cao 4, Gan Jiang 3, Fu Zi 2~3, Ren Shen 2

Tong Mai Si Ni Jia Zhu Dan Zhi Tang: Tong Mai Si Ni Tang + Zhu Dan 3

Gan Jiang Fu Zi Tang: Gan Jiang 6 + Fu Zi 6~9

Fu Zi Geng Mi Tang: Geng Mi 21, Ban Xia 12, Da Zao 5, Fu Zi 2~3, Gan Cao 2

Yi Yi Fu Zi San: Yi Yi Ren 30, Fu Zi 5~10

Yi Yi Fu Zi Bai Jiang San: Yi Yi Ren 20, Bai Jiang 10, Fu Zi 4

Bai Tong Tang: Cong Bai 6, Fu Zi 3~4.5, Gan Jiang 3

Bai Tong Jia Zhu Dan Zhi Tang: Bai Tong Tang + Zhu Dan Zhi 6, human urine 30

Da Wu Tou Jian: Wu Tou 10, honey 16

Wu Tou Tang: Ma Huang 6, Shao Yao 6, Huang Qi 6, Gan Cao 6 + Da Wu Tou Jian

Chi Wan: Fu Ling 8, Ban Xia 8, Wu Tou 4, Xi Xin 2

Zhen Wu Tang: Fu Ling 6, Shao Yao 6, Sheng Jiang 6, Zhu 4, Fu Zi 2~3

Fu Zi Tang: Zhu 8, Fu Ling 6, Shao Yao 6, Fu Zi 4~6, Ren Shen 4

Tian Xiong San: Zhu 16, Gui Zhi 12, Fu Zi 6, Long Gu 6

Zhi Zi / Xie Bai Formula Family

Zhi Zi Chi Tang: Xiang Chi 20, Zhi Zi 6

Zhi Zi Gan Cao Chi Tang: Zhi Zi Chi Tang + Gan Cao 6

Zhi Zi Sheng Jiang Chi Tang: Zhi Zi Chi Tang + Sheng Jiang 15

Zhi Shi Zhi Zi Chi Tang: Xiang Chi 32, Zhi Shi 6, Zhi Zi 4

Zhi Zi Da Huang Chi Tang: Xiang Chi 32, Zhi Shi 10, Zhi Zi 4, Da Huang 4

Yin Chen Hao Tang: Yin Chen Hao 12, Zhi Zi 4, Da Huang 4

Zhi Zi Bai Pi Tang: Zhi Zi 6, Huang Bai 6, Gan Cao 3

Zhi Zi Hou PoTang: Hou Po 8, Zhi Shi 8, Zhi Zi 4

Zhi Zi Gan Jiang Tang: Zhi Zi 6, Gan Jiang 6

Gua Lou Xie Bai Bai Jiu Tang: Xie Bai 24, Gua Lou Shi 6, Bai Jiu 420ml

Gua Lou Xie Bai Ban Xia Tang: Ban Xia 12, Xie Bai 6, Gua Lou Shi 4, Bai Jiu 400ml

Zhi Shi Xie Bai Gui Zhi Tang: Xie Bai 16, Zhi Shi 8, Hou Po 8, Gua Lou Shi 4, Gui Zhi 2

Huang Qin / Huang Lian / Ban Xia Formula Family

Da Ban Xia Tang: Ban Xia 48, Ren Shen 6, honey 16

Xiao Ban Xia Tang: Ban Xia 36, Sheng Jiang 24

Sheng Jiang Ban Xia Tang: Ban Xia 12, Sheng Jiang Zhi 40ml

Xiao Ban Xia Jia Fu Ling Tang: Xiao Ban Xia Tang + Fu Ling 9

Ban Xia Ku Jiu Tang: Ban Xia 5, Ku Jiu 35~40ml, egg shell 1 piece

Ban Xia Hou Po Tang: Ban Xia 24, Sheng Jiang 10, Fu Ling 8, Hou Po 6, Su Ye 4

Ban Xia Gan Jiang Tang: Ban Xia 1, Gan Jiang 1

Gan Jiang Ren Shen Ban Xia Wan: Ban Xia 2, Gan Jiang 1, Ren Shen 1

Ban Xia Xie Xin Tang: Ban Xia 12, Huang Qin 6, Gan Jiang 6, Ren Shen 6, Gan Cao 6, Da Zao 6, Huang Lian 2

Gan Cao Xi Xin Tang: Ban Xia Xie Xin Tang + Gan Cao 2

Sheng Jiang Xi Xin Tang: Ban Xia Xie Xin Tang + Sheng Jiang 8

Hou Po Sheng Jiang Ban Xia Gan Cao Ren Shen Tang: Hou Po 16, Sheng Jiang 16, Ban Xia 12, Gan Cao 4, Ren Shen 2

Huang Lian Tang: Ban Xia 12, Huang Lian 6, Gan Jiang 6, Gui Zhi 6, Da Zao 6, Gan Cao 6, Ren Shen 4

Gan Jiang Huang Qin Huang Lian Ren Shen Tang: Gan Jiang 9, Huang Qin 9, Huang Lian 9, Ren Shen 9

Da Jian Zhong Tang: Gan Jiang 8, Ren Shen 4, Chuan Jiao 3, Yi Tang 32

Huang Lian E Jiao Tang: Huang Lian 8, Shao Yao 4, Huang Qin 2, E Jiao 6, Ji Zi Huang 1

Huang Qin Tang: Huang Qin 6, Da Zao 6, Shao Yao 4, Gan Cao 4

Huang Qin Jia Ban Xia Sheng Jiang Tang: Huang Qin Tang + Ban Xia 12, Sheng Jiang 6

Liu Wu Huang Qin Tang: Ban Xia 12, Huang Qin 6, Ren Shen 6, Gan Jiang 6, Da Zao 6, Gui Zhi 4

San Wu Huang Qin Tang: Gan Di Huang 12, Ku Shen 6, Huang Qin 3

Bai Tou Weng Tang: Huang Lian 9, Huang Bai 9, Chen Pi 9, Bai Tou Weng 6

Bai Tou Weng Jia Gan Cao E Jiao Tang: Huang Lian 6, Huang Bai 6, Chen Pi 6, Bai Tou Weng 4, Gan Cao 4, E Jiao 4

Xiao Xian Xiong Tang: Ban Xia 12, Gua Lou Shi 8, Huang Lian 4

Xian Fu Hua Da Zhe Shi Tang: Ban Xia 12, Sheng Jiang 10, Ren Shen 6, Xian Fu Hua 6, Da Zao 6, Gan Cao 6, Da Zhe Shi 2

Mai Men Dong Tang: Mai Men Dong 30, Ban Xia 20, Geng Mi 12, Da Zao 6, Ren Shen 4, Gan Cao 4

Fang Ji / Zhi Shi / Ju Pi Formula Family

Mu Fang Ji Tang: Shi Gao 48, Ren Shen 8, Mu Fang Ji 6, Gui Zhi 4

Mu Fang Ji Qu Shi Gao Jia Fu Ling Mang Xiao Tang: Mu Fang Ji Tang – Shi Gao + Fu Ling 8 + Mang Xiao 8

Fang Ji Fu Ling Tang: Fu Ling 12, Fang Ji 6, Huang Qi 6, Gui Zhi 6, Gan Cao 4

Fang Ji Huang Qi Tang: Huang Qi 10, Fang Ji 8, Zhu 6, Da Zao 6, Sheng Jiang 6, Gan Cao 4

Zhi Shi Shao Yao San: Zhi Shi 6, Shao Yao 6

Zhi Zhu Tang: Zhi Shi 14, Zhu 4

Pai Nong San: Zhi Shi 12, Shao Yao 12, Jie Geng 4

Gui Zhi Sheng Jiang Zhi Shi Tang: Zhi Shi 10, Gui Zhi 6, Sheng Jiang 6

Ju Pi Zhi Shi Sheng Jiang Tang: Ju Pi 32, Sheng Jiang 16, Zhi Shi 6

Fu Ling Yin: Sheng Jiang 8, Fu Ling 6, Ren Shen 6, Zhu 6, Ju Pi 5, Zhi Shi 4

Ju Pi Zhu Ru Tang: Ju Pi 16, Sheng Jiang 16, Da Zao 15, Gan Cao 10, Zhu Ru 8, Ren Shen 2

Ju Pi Tang: Sheng Jiang 16, Ju Pi 8

Si Ni San: Chai Hu 6, Zhi Shi 6, Shao Yao 6, Gan Cao 6

Dang Gui / Chuan Xiong Formula Family

Xiong Gui Jiao Ai Tang: Gan Di Huang 12, Shao Yao 8, Ai Ye 6, Dang Gui 6, Chuan Xiong 4, E Jiao 4, Gan Cao 4

Wen Jing Tang: Mai Men Dong 10, Ban Xia 8, Dang Gui 4, Chuan Xiong 4, Shao Yao 4, Gui Zhi 4, E Jiao 4, Mu Dan Pi 4, Sheng Jiang 4, Gan Cao 4, Wu Zhu Yu 3

Dang Gui Shao Yao San: Shao Yao 16, Ze Xie 8, Fu Ling 4, Zhu 4, Dang Gui 3, Chuan Xiong 3

Dang Gui Si Ni Tang: Da Zao 12, Gui Zhi 6, Shao Yao 6, Dang Gui 6, Xi Xin 6, Mu Tong 4, Gan Cao 4

Dang Gui Si Ni Jia Wu Zhu Yu Sheng Jiang Tang: Sheng Jiang 15, Da Zao 12, Gui Zhi 6, Shao Yao 6, Dang Gui 6, Xi Xin 6, Wu Zhu Yu 4, Mu Tong 4, Gan Cao 4

Dang Gui Gan Zhong Tang: Shao Yao 12, Dang Gui 8, Gui Zhi 6, Sheng Jiang 6, Da Zao 6, Gan Cao 4

Dang Gui San: Dang Gui 16, Huang Qin 16, Shao Yao 16, Chuan Xiong 16, Zhu 8

Bai Zhu San: Bai Zhu 6, Chuan Xiong 6, Chuan Jiao 6, Mu Li 4

Other Formulas

Wu Zhu Yu Tang: Wu Zhu Yu 5, Sheng Jiang 6, Da Zao 4, Ren Shen 3

Ren Shen Tang: Ren Shen 6, Gan Jiang 6, Zhu 6, Gan Cao 6

Ting Li Da Zao Xie Fei Tang: Da Zao 18, Ting Li 6

Ma Zi Ren Wan: Ma Zi Ren 10, Da Huang 8, Zhi Shi 8, Xing Ren 6, Hou Po 4, Shao Yao 4

Shi Zao Tang: Da Zao 12, Gan Sui 0.7, Da Ji 0.7, Yuan Hua 0.7

Jie Geng Bai San: Jieng Geng 3, Bei Mu 3, Ba Dou 1

Zou Ma Tang: Ba Dou 2, Xing Ren 2

Suan Zao Ren Tang: Suan Zao Ren 48, Zhi Mu 4, Fu Ling 4, Chuan Xiong 4, Gan Cao 2

Bibliography

Dr. Song Il-Byung, <An introduction to Sasang Constitutional Medicine> Seoul: Jipmoondang International, 2005

Dr. Kang Joobong, <The dynamics of Shang Han Lun>, published by IOMRI

Kim Jongyeol and Duong Duc Pham, <Sasang Constitutional Medicine as a Holistic Tailored Medicine>

Sasang Constitutional Medicine, published by Jip Moon Dang (Korean Version)

Dr. Kuon Dowon, <Eight Constitutional Medicine : An overview>, Institute for Modern Korean Studies, 2003

Lee Gangjae, <The practice of Eight Constitutional Medicine>, Haeng Lim Seo Won 2009 (Korean version)

CMC research group, <The heavenly regimen>, Korea Medical, 2004 (Korean version)

Hiromichi Yasui, <Medical History in Japan>, The Journal of Kampo, Japan Institute of TCM Research, 2007

Lee Junghuan and Jung Changhyun, <Yakucho of Todo Yoshimasu>, Chung Hong, 2006 (Korean version)

Yumoto Kyushin, <Japanese-Chinese Medicine (Kokan Igaku)(Huang Han Yi Xue)>, Gye Chuk Moon Hwa Sa, 2015 (Korean version)

Otsuka Keisetsu, <The Interpretation of Shang Han Lun> transtlated by Park Byunghee, Eui Bang, 2015 (Korean version)

Craig Mitchelle, Feng Ye, Nigel Wiseman, <Shang Han Lun>, Paradigm Publications

Philippe Sionneau &Lu Gang, <The treatment of Disease in TCM>, Blue Poppy Press, 2000

Otsuka Keisetsu, <Shang Han Lun: Wellspring of Chinese Medicine> edited by Hong Yen Hsu, William G. Pitcher, Keats Publishing, 1981

Jun-Su Jang, Young-Su Kim, Boncho Ku, and Jong Yeol Kim,<Recent Progress in Voice-Based Sasang Constitutional Medicine: Improving Stability of Diagnosis>

Eunsu Jang, Jong Yeol Kim, Haejung Lee, Honggie Kim, Younghwa Baek, and Siwoo Lee,<A Study on the Reliability of Sasang Constitutional Body Trunk Measurement

http://www.hindawi.com/journals

Evidence-Based Complementary and Alternative Medicine
Volume 2014 (2014), Article ID 740515, 6 pages
http://dx.doi.org/10.1155/2014/740515
<Introduction to the History and Current Status of Evidence-Based Korean Medicine: A Unique Integrated System of Allopathic and Holistic Medicine>
Chang Shik Yin and Seong-Gyu Ko
http://www.hindawi.com/journals/ecam/2013/920384/

Evidence-Based Complementary and Alternative Medicine
Volume 2013 (2013), Article ID 920384, 7 pages
http://dx.doi.org/10.1155/2013/920384

Evidence-Based Complementary and Alternative Medicine
Volume 2013 (2013), Article ID 920384, 7 pages
http://dx.doi.org/10.1155/2013/920384

Evidence-Based Complementary and Alternative Medicine
Volume 2012 (2012), Article ID 604842, 8 pages
http://dx.doi.org/10.1155/2012/604842

Evidence-Based Complementary and Alternative Medicine
Volume 2014 (2014), Article ID 535146, 5 pages
http://dx.doi.org/10.1155/2014/535146 Pattern Classification in Kampo Medicine
by S. Yakubo, M. Ito, Y. Ueda, H. Okamoto, Y. Kimura, Y. Amano, T. Togo, H.
Adachi, T. Mitsuma, and K. Watanabe

https://en.wikipedia.org/wiki/Kampo

https://en.wikipedia.org/wiki/Shanghan_Lun

Acknowledgement

First of all, I would like to convey my gratitude to the senior Traditional Asian Medicine practitioners who have built theoretical foundation of herbology and formula writing and have translated and interpreted the old text into the modern version. I would also like to thank my families for their unconditional love, support, and trust. Last but not least, I would like to express my gratitude to my English tutor, Matthew Serrins, who reviewed and corrected each sentence of my writing. This book could not be completed without his help.